HEALTH CARE COSTS FOR CONSUMERS, SMALL BUSINESSES AND THE BUREAU OF PRISONS

Small Business Considerations, Economics and Research

Additional books and e-books in this series can be found on Nova's website under the Series tab.

Health Care in Transition

Additional books and e-books in this series can be found on Nova's website under the Series tab.

SMALL BUSINESS CONSIDERATIONS, ECONOMICS AND RESEARCH

HEALTH CARE COSTS FOR CONSUMERS, SMALL BUSINESSES AND THE BUREAU OF PRISONS

MAIK NACHT
EDITOR

New York

NOTICE TO THE READER

The Publisher has taken reasonable care in the preparation of this book, but makes no expressed or implied warranty of any kind and assumes no responsibility for any errors or omissions. No liability is assumed for incidental or consequential damages in connection with or arising out of information contained in this book. The Publisher shall not be liable for any special, consequential, or exemplary damages resulting, in whole or in part, from the readers' use of, or reliance upon, this material. Any parts of this book based on government reports are so indicated and copyright is claimed for those parts to the extent applicable to compilations of such works.

Independent verification should be sought for any data, advice or recommendations contained in this book. In addition, no responsibility is assumed by the Publisher for any injury and/or damage to persons or property arising from any methods, products, instructions, ideas or otherwise contained in this publication.

This publication is designed to provide accurate and authoritative information with regard to the subject matter covered herein. It is sold with the clear understanding that the Publisher is not engaged in rendering legal or any other professional services. If legal or any other expert assistance is required, the services of a competent person should be sought. FROM A DECLARATION OF PARTICIPANTS JOINTLY ADOPTED BY A COMMITTEE OF THE AMERICAN BAR ASSOCIATION AND A COMMITTEE OF PUBLISHERS.

Additional color graphics may be available in the e-book version of this book.

Library of Congress Cataloging-in-Publication Data

ISBN: 978-1-53616-862-4

Published by Nova Science Publishers, Inc. † New York

Contents

PREFACE

Healthcare costs continue to rise in the United States and many Americans are struggling to budget and pay for their healthcare expenses. As healthcare costs continue to rise, many Americans still have no idea how much something will cost them before they receive care. Chapter 1 examines some of the causes of increased healthcare costs, and increasing healthcare costs.

One of the biggest challenges for small businesses wishing to help their employees with health care is the cost. Small businesses helping their employees purchase health insurance is discussed in chapter 2.

From fiscal years 2009 through 2016, the Bureau of Prisons (BOP) obligated more than $9 billion for the provision of inmate health care and several factors affected these costs. Chapter 3 addresses BOP's costs to provide health care services and factors that affect costs; the extent to which BOP has data to help control health care costs; and the extent to which BOP has planned and implemented cost control efforts.

Chapter 1 - This is an edited, reformatted and augmented version of Hearing before the Subcommittee on Oversight and Investigations of the Committee on Energy and Commerce, House of Representatives, One Hundred Fifteenth Congress, Second Session, Publication No. Serial No. 115–151, dated July 17, 2018.

Chapter 2 - This is an edited, reformatted and augmented version of Hearing Before the Subcommittee on Primary Health and Retirement Security of the Committee on Health, Education, Labor, and Pensions United States Senate, One Hundred Fourteenth Congress, Second Session, Publication No. S. HRG. 114–782, dated 2018.

Chapter 3 - As of June 2017, BOP was responsible for the custody and care—including health care—of about 154,000 inmates housed in BOP institutions. Health care includes medical, dental, and psychological treatment. BOP provides most care inside its institutions, but transports inmates outside when circumstances warrant. GAO was asked to review health care costs at BOP institutions.

This report addresses: (1) BOP's costs to provide health care services and factors that affect costs; (2) the extent to which BOP has data to help control health care costs; and (3) the extent to which BOP has planned and implemented cost control efforts.

GAO analyzed BOP health care obligations data for fiscal years 2009 through 2016, gathered information on BOP's health care cost control initiatives through a data collection instrument, and reviewed BOP's health care related strategic plans. GAO also interviewed BOP officials and visited 10 BOP institutions, selected in part, for total and per capita medical services costs.

In: Health Care Costs for Consumers ... ISBN: 978-1-53616-862-4
Editor: Maik Nacht

Chapter 1

EXAMINING STATE EFFORTS TO IMPROVE TRANSPARENCY OF HEALTHCARE COSTS FOR CONSUMERS*

Subcommittee on Oversight and Investigations

Tuesday, July 17, 2018
House of Representatives,
Subcommittee on Oversight and Investigations,
Committee on Energy and Commerce, *Washington, DC.*

The subcommittee met, pursuant to call, at 10:15 a.m., in room 2322 Rayburn House Office Building, Hon. Gregg Harper (chairman of the subcommittee) presiding.

Members present: Representatives Harper, Griffith, Barton, Burgess, Brooks, Collins, Walberg, Walters, Costello, Carter, Walden (ex officio),

* This is an edited, reformatted and augmented version of Hearing before the Subcommittee on Oversight and Investigations of the Committee on Energy and Commerce, House of Representatives, One Hundred Fifteenth Congress, Second Session, Publication No. Serial No. 115–151, dated July 17, 2018.

DeGette, Schakowsky, Castor, Tonko, Clarke, Ruiz, and Pallone (ex officio).

Staff present: Jennifer Barblan, Chief Counsel, Oversight & Investigations; Lamar Echols, Counsel, Oversight & Investigations; Ali Fulling, Legislative Clerk, Oversight & Investigations, Digital Commerce and Consumer Protection; Jennifer Sherman, Press Secretary; Austin Stonebraker, Press Assistant; Hamlin Wade, Special Advisor, External Affairs; Jeff Carroll, Minority Staff Director; Chris Knauer, Minority Oversight Staff Director; Miles Lichtman, Minority Policy Analyst; Kevin McAloon, Minority Professional Staff Member; C.J. Young, Minority Press Secretary; and Perry Lusk, Minority GAO Detailee.

OPENING STATEMENT OF HON. GREGG HARPER, A REPRESENTATIVE IN CONGRESS FROM THE STATE OF MISSISSIPPI

Mr. HARPER. I call to order the hearing of the subcommittee on Oversight and Investigations.

Today, the Subcommittee on Oversight and Investigations is holding a hearing entitled, "Examining State Efforts to Improve Transparency of Healthcare Costs for Consumers." We are here today because healthcare costs continue to rise in the United States and many Americans are struggling to budget and pay for their healthcare expenses.

According to the Centers for Medicare and Medicaid Services, we spent $3.3 trillion on healthcare costs in 2016, which means that nearly 18 percent of the overall share of gross domestic product was related to healthcare spending. About 32 percent of healthcare spending in 2016 was on hospital care, 20 percent was on physician and clinical services, and about 10 percent of the spending was on prescription drugs.

The Committee has been actively looking at these concerning trends and has held a number of hearings examining some of the causes of increased healthcare costs, and increasing healthcare costs. Last year, the

Oversight and Investigations subcommittee held two hearings on the 340B Drug Pricing Program and issued a report with the findings from our investigations. In February, the subcommittee held a hearing examining consolidation in the healthcare market, and examined the impact of consolidation on healthcare competition and innovation.

As healthcare costs continue to rise, many Americans still have no idea how much something will cost them before they receive care. Oftentimes, they only know their out-of-pocket costs once they have gotten the care and get their bill weeks, sometimes months later. The purpose of today's hearing is to examine state laws and policies that have an impact on healthcare costs and what can be done to lower costs for all Americans through more transparency of healthcare costs.

These transparency efforts have generally attempted to provide consumers information about different types of healthcare costs, including information about the cost of healthcare services and the cost of prescription drugs. In our work, we have heard that there are a number of issues that make it difficult for some of these efforts to be effective.

For example, sometimes there may be contractual provisions that limit the sharing of certain price information or concerns that the sharing of certain price information may be anti-competitive. Moreover, healthcare billing is complex and it can be difficult to provide the information to consumers in a meaningful way that is useful to them. Similarly, only a small percentage of healthcare services may be "shoppable." I hope to hear more about some of the barriers to transparency and what, if anything, Congress can do to help.

Unfortunately, early evidence suggests that some price transparency tools have not helped facilitate price shopping and lower consumer costs. I, therefore, look forward to hearing more from the witnesses about why this is the case, and what forms of transparency might help consumers as they budget for their care and make better healthcare decisions. For example, do we need to pair transparency with some other mechanism for it to be most effective?

The cost of certain healthcare services can vary significantly in the same geographic region at different sites of care. For instance, a 2014 study by the U.S. Government Accountability Office found that the estimated cost of maternity care at select, high-quality acute care hospitals in the Boston area ranged between $6,834 and $21,554, over a 200 percent difference.

A more recent 2018 study found that median price of magnetic resonance imaging, an MRI, of the spine ranges from $500 to $1,670 in Massachusetts, also over a 200 percent difference.

Empowering consumers with more information about the cost and quality of their care helps to reduce wasteful spending and save families money.

As we move forward, we have to keep in mind that there is a delicate balance between beneficial transparency and transparency that ultimately harms competition and consumers. The Federal Trade Commission has highlighted that it is important to give consumers the precise information they need to make better healthcare decisions. The agency also has cautioned, however, that it is important to avoid broad disclosures that may chill competition in the healthcare market.

I welcome and thank the witnesses for being here today. I look forward to their testimony.

And I will now recognize Ms. Castor for purposes of an opening statement.

[The prepared statement of Mr. Harper follows:]

PREPARED STATEMENT OF HON. GREGG HARPER

Today, the Subcommittee on Oversight and Investigations is holding a hearing entitled, "Examining State Efforts to Improve Transparency of Healthcare Costs for Consumers." We are here because healthcare costs continue to rise in the United States and many Americans are struggling to budget and pay for their healthcare expenses.

According to the Centers for Medicare and Medicaid Services, we spent $3.3 trillion on healthcare in 2016, which means nearly 18 percent of the overall share of gross domestic product was related to healthcare spending. About 32 percent of healthcare spending in 2016 was on hospital care, 20 percent was on physician and clinical services, and about 10 percent of the spending was on prescription drugs. The Committee has been actively looking at this concerning trend and has held a number of hearings examining some of the causes of increasing healthcare costs. Last year, the Oversight and Investigations subcommittee held two hearings on the 340B Drug Pricing Program and issued a report with the findings from our investigation. In February, the subcommittee held a hearing examining consolidation in the healthcare market and examined the impact of consolidation on healthcare competition and innovation.

As healthcare costs continue to rise, many Americans still have no idea how much something will cost them before they receive care. Oftentimes, they only know their out of pocket costs once they have gotten the care and get their bill weeks, sometimes months, later. The purpose of today's hearing is to examine state laws and policies that have an impact on healthcare costs and what can be done to lower costs for all Americans through more transparency of healthcare costs.

These transparency efforts have generally attempted to provide consumers information about different types of healthcare costs, including information about the cost of healthcare services and the cost of prescription drugs. In our work, we've heard that there are a number of issues that make it difficult for some of these efforts to be effective. For example, sometimes there may be contractual provisions that limit the sharing of certain price information or concerns that the sharing of certain price information may be anti-competitive. Moreover, healthcare billing is complex and it can be difficult to provide the information to consumers in a meaningful way that is useful to them. Similarly, only a small percentage of healthcare services may be "shoppable." I hope to hear more about some of the barriers to transparency and what, if anything, Congress can do to help.

Unfortunately, early evidence suggests that some price transparency tools have not helped facilitate price shopping and lower consumer costs. I therefore look forward to hearing more from the witnesses about why this is the case, and what forms of transparency might help consumers budget for their care and make better healthcare decisions. For example, do we need to pair transparency with some other mechanism for it to be most effective?

The cost of certain healthcare services can vary significantly in the same geographic region at different sites of care. For instance, a 2014 study by the U.S. Government Accountability Office found that the estimated cost of maternity care at select, high-quality acute care hospitals in the Boston area ranged between $6,834 and $21,554—over a 100 percent difference. A more recent 2018 study found that the median price of magnetic resonance imaging (MRI) of the spine ranges from $500 to $1,670 in Massachusetts-also over a 100 percent difference. Empowering consumers with more information about the cost and quality of their care could help to reduce wasteful spending and save families money.

As we move forward, we have to keep in mind that there is a delicate balance between beneficial transparency and transparency that ultimately harms competition and consumers. The Federal Trade Commission has highlighted that it is important to give consumers the precise information they need to make better healthcare decisions. The agency also has cautioned, however, that it is important to avoid broad disclosures that may chill competition in the healthcare market.

I welcome and thank the witnesses for being here today, and I look forward to their testimony.

OPENING STATEMENT OF HON. KATHY CASTOR, A REPRESENTATIVE IN CONGRESS FROM THE STATE OF FLORIDA

Ms. CASTOR. Well, thank you, Mr. Chairman. Thank you for calling this important hearing. I think it is a worthy topic.

But, I wanted to note at the outset it has been almost 1 month since the Democrats on this committee have requested an oversight hearing on the Administration's family separation policy. The Energy and Commerce

Committee has primary responsibility for oversight of the Department of Health and Human Services. We have had over the last month a number of hearings on many varied topics, but none are as important as what is happening as children who are ripped away from their family. Now, courts have ordered reunification.

It is our responsibility as Members of Congress, especially in the Oversight Committee of Energy and Commerce, to have an oversight hearing to get to the bottom of this. We hear horrifying stories every day about the impact on children.

And so at this time I am going to renew the request of the Democrats on Energy and Commerce to schedule an oversight hearing as soon as possible on the family separation policy.

Now, healthcare costs, also a very worthy topic. And if we were to schedule another important oversight hearing, it certainly should be on the impact of the Trump administration's lawsuit that where they claim that preexisting conditions should not be a right of American families, especially in their healthcare policy. That would be another very worthy oversight hearing. But, right now we are here on transparency, so let's talk about that.

I understand that every family feels a very significant impact of rising prices. And part of the problem is the fact that healthcare consumers often have no visibility into how much services are actually going to cost.

And depending on multiple factors, such as where you live, your insurance, the type of provider, costs can vary greatly and are unpredictable. That makes healthcare unlike virtually any other purchase, and it makes it more difficult to constrain costs.

There are all sorts of reports out there—many of you all have experienced this—of outrageously high bills received by unsuspecting consumers. Plus, it is darn confusing sometimes. You get a bill and it says this is your responsibility, this is what is paid, and people simply don't, don't, get it.

There was a couple in California recently who were reportedly charged over $18,000 for a 3-hour visit to an emergency room where their baby was examined, took a nap, and drank formula. And another patient received two CT scans that varied between $268 and $9,000.

These shockingly high bills are frustrating and can devastate a family's finances. For that reason, greater transparency can theoretically provide consumers with more information to make decisions and to predict the costs that they are going to incur.

To that end, many states have taken some action to bring more transparency to healthcare. But it isn't always easy. My home State of Florida, for example, established a website that allows consumers to search for healthcare prices at hospitals and outpatient surgery centers in 2007, but consumers don't know about it. And one of the problems is it doesn't even contain all of the hospitals that are in your market, and it doesn't contain a lot of the leading health insurers' information in our state.

So there, Florida is currently struggling with trying to launch another healthcare transparency website but now the cost is really escalating. It has been $4 million to get that up and running, and we don't have a lot to show for it.

Other states now require pharmaceutical companies to publicize and provide information related to large increases in prices for certain drugs. And here in the House I am a proud cosponsor of Congresswoman Schakowsky's Fair Accountability and Innovative Research Drug Pricing Act, which would require drug companies to report an increase in certain drug prices by more than 10 percent in a year to HHS, and submit transparency and justification reports before they increase the price of certain drugs by 10 percent.

We should move initiatives that can help consumers control their healthcare costs. But transparency in our healthcare system shouldn't be the only tool in our tool box. It has to be accompanied with other improvements to have a meaningful impact on the actual cost of care.

So, I am looking forward to hearing the witnesses today. I look forward to hearing from you on how we can use healthcare transparency to lower costs for our neighbors back home.

Thank you, and I yield back.

[The prepared statement of Ms. Castor follows:]

PREPARED STATEMENT OF HON. KATHY CASTOR

Thank you, Mr. Chairman. Healthcare costs continue to account for a large portion of our economy, and every family feels the impact of rising prices. Part of this problem is the fact that healthcare consumers often have no visibility into how much services are actually going to cost.

Depending on multiple factors such as the geographical area, a patient's insurance, and the type of provider, costs can vary greatly and seem unpredictable to the consumer. That makes healthcare unlike virtually any other commodity, and makes it more difficult to constrain costs.

We have seen news reports of outrageously high bills received by unsuspecting consumers. There was the couple in California who were reportedly charged over $18,000 for a 3-hour visit to an emergency room, where their baby was examined, took a nap, and drank formula. And another patient received two CT scans that varied between $268 and nearly $9,000.

These shocking bills are frustrating and can devastate a family's finances. For that reason, greater transparency can theoretically provide consumers with more information to make decisions and predict the costs they are going to incur.

To that end, many states have taken some action to bring more transparency to healthcare. My home State of Florida, for example, established a website that allows consumers to search for healthcare prices at hospitals and outpatient surgery centers. Other states now require pharmaceutical companies to publicize and provide information related to large increases in prices for certain drugs.

These efforts are well-intended, and we should applaud any initiative that has the potential to help consumers control their healthcare costs. That being said, we also must keep in mind that transparency is not a panacea, and must be coupled with other improvements to have a meaningful impact on the actual cost of care.

As we will hear from the witnesses today, transparency initiatives by themselves are not tremendously effective at bringing down consumer healthcare costs. What sounds like a straightforward solution in most markets does not always work in healthcare, for multiple reasons.

For one thing, when people's health is at stake, information on prices might not be relevant. People naturally trust their doctor and want the best care. And when we see greater consolidation in the healthcare industry, transparency cannot provide much help to consumers with no leverage to access lower prices.

So we need to consider what the research says: what types of transparency reforms can work, what does not work, and how transparency needs to be combined with more meaningful actions.

For instance, Mr. Chairman, a key part of bringing down costs for consumers is ensuring access to high-quality and affordable healthcare, including primary care. We need to give consumers more than just information—we need to bring relief from these rising costs in the first place. Without that, these transparency efforts will be in vain, and we'll just be shining a spotlight on continuously increasing costs. That is not to say that transparency does not have a role. Instead, we should look to combine transparency initiatives with incentives to provide higher quality care at lower costs. I hope to hear the witnesses' perspective on that today.

I thank the witnesses for being here today, and I yield back.

Mr. HARPER. The gentlewoman yields back.

The chair will now recognize the chairman of the full committee,

Mr. Walden, for 5 minutes.

Opening Statement of Hon. Greg Walden, a Representative in Congress from the State of Oregon

Mr. WALDEN. Thank you very much, Mr. Chairman. I appreciate your holding this hearing on the various transparency efforts at the state level to engage patients in healthcare decision making processes.

As Chairman Harper mentioned in his opening statement, healthcare costs are increasing and are expected to continue to rise. In 2016, the U.S. spent approximately $3.3 trillion on healthcare, and the Center for Medicare and Medicaid Services, CMS, estimates that spending will reach $5.7 trillion in 2026.

Healthcare costs are having a substantial impact on the budgets of American families and individuals. In addition to health insurance premiums increasing, patients are also directly responsible for more of their healthcare costs. In 2016, about 11 percent of the $3.3 trillion spent on healthcare was paid for directly by consumers through out-of-pocket costs, which was about $352 billion.

Unsurprisingly, as healthcare costs increase, most patients want to know more about how much different medical services and products are going to cost them. We all do. That is why we are having this hearing. I have heard numerous stories about individuals who were going to have a medical procedure or lab work performed, found it nearly impossible, and in some instances literally impossible, to learn how much it was going to cost them before they got the care. A lot of doctors don't even know how much different services are going to cost.

Many states have adopted policies to prohibit some types of "gag clauses" and help patients get access to the prices for prescription drugs. Twenty-two states have passed legislation prohibiting clauses in contracts that prohibit pharmacists from telling patients price options for their prescription medicine.

In addition to these recent efforts to encourage price information sharing with patients at the pharmacy counter, several states have engaged in efforts to provide patients with more information about the price and quality of different healthcare services. Some of these efforts include creating websites that give patients information about the prices of different procedures, requiring insurers to provide these tools to their members, and requiring providers to give patients information about the estimated prices for their treatment before they get the treatment. Unfortunately, to date, some of the preliminary evidence has shown that these tools haven't been very effective in getting patients to price shop.

If we are going to successfully reduce healthcare costs, we need to empower patients and we need to engage them in the decision-making process. So there needs to be greater transparency so patients can have more information about the prices for different medical products and services, and that information needs to be given to them in a meaningful way.

Given that some of the existing price transparency tools are still able to be improved, I am eager to hear from our witnesses today about why there are some of these barriers, and then also what else we can do to empower patients with the information. I also want to hear about the role the Federal Government can play in promoting transparency and making patients more informed about the cost of their care.

Patients should be able to learn about how much something is going to cost before they get it. This includes having information about different price options for prescription drugs at the pharmacy counter, and information about different procedures and lab work, among other things.

So, we have got a lot of questions for our witnesses today. We really appreciate your being here. But one of my main questions is what is the best way for patients to get healthcare price information, and how can we empower the consumer?

I am also interested in hearing about any market behaviors that work against transparency and ultimately harm any attempts to bring down healthcare costs.

So, thanks for being here. This is a big priority for me and for the committee to look into all the costs of healthcare.

With that I will just warn you, I have got another hearing going on downstairs so I have to bounce back and forth. But I will yield the balance of my time to Dr. Burgess, who chairs our Health Subcommittee.

[The prepared statement of Mr. Walden follows:]

PREPARED STATEMENT OF HON. GREG WALDEN

Thank you, Mr. Chairman, for holding this hearing on the various transparency efforts at the state level to engage patients in the healthcare decision-making process.

As Chairman Harper mentioned in his opening statement, healthcare costs are increasing and are expected to continue to rise. In 2016, the U.S. spent approximately $3.3 trillion on healthcare, and the Centers for Medicare and Medicaid Services (CMS) estimates that spending will reach $5.7 trillion by 2026.

Healthcare costs are having a substantial impact on the budgets of American families and individuals. In addition to health insurance premiums increasing, patients are also directly responsible for more of their healthcare costs. In 2016, about 11 percent of the $3.3 trillion spent on healthcare was paid for directly by consumers through out-of-pocket costs-which was about $352 billion dollars.

Unsurprisingly, as healthcare costs increase, most patients want to know more about how much different medical services and products are going to cost them. We all do. I've heard numerous stories about individuals who were going to have a medical procedure or lab work performed and found it nearly impossible, and in some instances impossible, to learn how much it was going to cost them before they got the care. A lot of doctors don't even know how much different services are going to cost.

Many states have adopted policies to prohibit some types of "gag clauses" and help patients get access to the prices for prescription drugs. Twenty-two states have passed legislation prohibiting clauses in contracts that prohibit pharmacists from telling patients price options for their prescription medicine.

In addition to these recent efforts to encourage price information sharing with patients at the pharmacy counter, several states have engaged in efforts to provide patients with more information about the price and quality of different healthcare services. Some of these efforts include creating websites that give patients information about the prices of different procedures, requiring insurers to provide these tools to their members, and requiring providers to give patients information about the estimated prices for their treatment before they get the treatment. Unfortunately, to date, some of the preliminary evidence has shown that these some of these tools haven't been very effective in getting patients to price shop.

If we're going to successfully reduce healthcare costs, we need to empower patients and engage them in the decision-making process. There needs to be greater transparency, so patients can have more information about the prices for different medical products and services, and that information needs to be given to them in a meaningful way.

Given that some of the existing price transparency tools are still able to be improved, I'm eager to hear from the witnesses today about why there are some of these barriers and then also what else we can be doing to empower patients with information. I also want to hear about the role that the federal government can play in promoting transparency and making patients more informed about the cost of their care.

Patients should be able to learn about how much something is going to cost them before they get it. This includes having information about different price options for prescription drugs at the pharmacy counter and information about different procedures and lab work, among other things.

I have a lot of questions for the witnesses today, but one of my main questions is what is the best way for patients to be getting healthcare price information and how can we help empower patients? I also am interested in hearing about any market behaviors that work against transparency and ultimately harm any attempts to bring down healthcare costs.

I'd like to thank our witnesses for being with us today, and look forward to their feedback on those questions and others. There is clearly a lot to be discussed in regards to today's topic, and I look forward to a robust dialogue.

Mr. BURGESS. Well, thank you, Mr. Chairman. And, Mr. Chairman, it is my fondest wish that one day I will come into a hearing in the Energy and Commerce Committee and there will be five doctors at the witness table, and they are going to expound for us on how much economists should be paid. I am still waiting for that hearing. We haven't had it yet.

Thanks to our witnesses for being here today. And, Mr. Chairman, to you I have a couple of things that I would just like to place into the record.

This is a copy of H.R. 5547, a bill that was introduced in the last Congress by Mr. Green and I that dealt with transparency. And, in fact, Mr. Green and I have been working on transparency for the past several years. And a version of this was actually included as an amendment in the Affordable Care Act, but I think it got lost on its way to the Senate.

Mr. HARPER. Without objection.

[The information follows:]

H. R. 5547, 114TH CONGRESS, 2ND SESSION

To amend title XIX of the Social Security Act to provide for increased price transparency of hospital information and to provide for additional research on consumer information on charges and out-of-pocket costs.

In the House of Representatives, June 21, 2016

Mr. BURGESS (for himself and Mr. GENE GREEN of Texas) introduced the following bill; which was referred to the Committee on Energy and Commerce.

A Bill

To amend title XIX of the Social Security Act to provide for increased price transparency of hospital information and to provide for additional research on consumer information on charges and out-of-pocket costs.

Be it enacted by the Senate and House of Representatives of the United States of America in Congress assembled,

Section 1. Short Title

This Act may be cited as the "Health Care Price Transparency Promotion Act of 2016."

Sec. 2. Increasing the Transparency of Information on Hospital Charges and Making Available Information on Estimated Out-of-Pocket Costs for Health Care Services

(a) IN GENERAL.—Title XIX of the Social Security

Act is amended—

(1) in section 1902(a) (42 U.S.C. 1396a(a)), by inserting after paragraph (77) the following new paragraph:

"(78) provide that the State will establish and maintain laws, in accordance with the requirements of section 1921A, to require disclosure of information on hospital charges, to make such information available to the public, and to provide individuals with information about estimated out-of-pocket costs for health care services;" and

(2) by inserting after section 1921 (42 U.S.C. 1396r–2) the following new section:

"INCREASING THE TRANSPARENCY OF INFORMATION ON HOSPITAL CHARGES AND PROVIDING CONSUMERS WITH ESTIMATES OF OUT-OF-POCKET COSTS FOR HEALTH CARE SERVICES

"SEC. 1921A. (a) IN GENERAL.—The requirements referred to in section 1902(a)(78) are that the laws of a State must—

"(1) in accordance with subsection (b)—

"(A) require the disclosure of information on hospital charges; and

"(B) provide for access to such information; and

"(2) in accordance with subsection (c), require the provision of a statement of the estimated out-of-pocket costs of an individual for anticipated future health care services.

"(b) INFORMATION ON HOSPITAL CHARGES.—The laws of a State must—

"(1) require disclosure, by each hospital located in the State, of information on the charges for certain inpatient and outpatient hospital services (as determined by the State) provided at the hospital; and

"(2) provide for timely access to such information by individuals seeking or requiring such services.

"(c) Estimated Out-of-Pocket Costs.—The laws of a State must require that, upon the request of any individual with health insurance coverage sponsored by a health insurance issuer, the issuer must provide a statement of the estimated out-of-pocket costs that are likely to be incurred by the individual if the individual receives particular health care items and services within a specified period of time.

"(d) RULES OF CONSTRUCTION.—Nothing in this section shall be construed as—

"(1) authorizing or requiring the Secretary to establish uniform standards for the State laws required by subsections (b) and (c);

"(2) requiring any State with a law enacted on or before the date of the enactment of this section that—

"(A) meets the requirements of subsection (b) or subsection (c) to modify or amend such law; or

"(B) meets some but not all of the requirements of subsection (b) or subsection (c) to modify or amend such law except to the extent necessary to address the unmet requirements;

"(3) precluding any State in which a program of voluntary disclosure of information on hospital charges is in effect from adopting a law codifying such program (other than its voluntary nature) to satisfy the requirement of subsection (b)(1); or

"(4) guaranteeing that the out-of-pocket costs of an individual will not exceed the estimate of such costs provided pursuant to subsection (c).

"(e) DEFINITIONS.—For purposes of this section:

"(1) The term 'health insurance coverage' has the meaning given such term in section 2791(b)(1) of the Public Health Service Act.

"(2) The term 'health insurance issuer' has the meaning given such term in section 2791(b)(2) of the Public Health Service Act, except that such term also includes—

"(A) a Medicaid managed care organization (as defined in section 1903(m)); and

"(B) a Medicare Advantage organization (as defined in section 1859(a)(1), taking into account the operation of section 201(b) of the Medicare Prescription Drug, Improvement, and Modernization Act of 2003).

Section 1856(b)(3) shall not preclude the application to a Medicare Advantage organization or a Medicare Advantage plan offered by such an organization of any State law adopted to carry out the requirements of subsection (b) or (c).

"(3) The term 'hospital' means an institution that meets the requirements of paragraphs (1) and (7) of section 1861(e) and includes those to which section 1820(c) applies."

(b) EFFECTIVE DATE.—

(1) IN GENERAL.—Except as provided in paragraph (2), the amendments made by subsection (a) shall take effect on October 1, 2017.

(2) EXCEPTION.—In the case of a State plan for medical assistance under title XIX of the Social Security Act which the Secretary of Health and Human Services determines requires State legislation (other than legislation appropriating funds) in order for the plan to meet the additional requirements imposed by the amendment made by subsection (a), the State plan shall not be regarded as failing to comply with the requirements of such title solely on the basis of its failure to meet these additional requirements before the first day of the first calendar quarter beginning after the close of the first regular session of the State legislature that begins after the date of the enactment of this Act. For purposes of the previous sentence, in the case of a State that has a 2-year legislative session, each year of such session shall be deemed to be a separate regular session of the State legislature.

Sec. 3. Research on Information Valued by Consumers on Charges and out-of-Pocket Costs for Health Care Services

(a) RESEARCH ON INFORMATION VALUED AND USED BY CONSUMERS.—The Director of the Agency for Healthcare Research and Quality (in this section referred to as "AHRQ") shall conduct or support research, pursuant to section 901(b)(1)(D) of the Public Health Service 9 Act (42 U.S.C. 299(b)(1)(D)), on—

(1) the types of information on the charges, and out-of-pocket costs, for health care services that individuals find useful in making decisions about where, when, and from whom to receive care;

(2) how the types of information valued by individuals for making such decisions vary by whether they have health benefits coverage and, if they do, the type of such coverage they have, such as traditional insurance, health maintenance organizations, preferred provider organizations, and high deductible plans coupled with health savings accounts; and

(3) ways in which such information may be made available on a timely basis and in easy-to-understand form to individuals facing such decisions.

(b) REPORT.—The Director of AHRQ shall report to the Congress on the results of such research not later than 18 months after the date of the enactment of this Act, together with recommendations for ways in which the Federal Government can assist the States in achieving the objective specified in subsection (a)(3).

(c) AUTHORIZATION OF APPROPRIATIONS.—There are authorized to be appropriated such sums as may be necessary to carry out this section.

Mr. BURGESS. Also, I would like to place for the record, I printed off some sheets from a website called txpricepoint.org. Texas PricePoint is a website that is at the least sponsored by the Texas Hospital Association, and it is useful information for your county or for your city, for the hospital in your county or for your city.

For example, I printed off a sheet that I will, I will leave for the record that deals with the cost of an uncomplicated cesarean section in the hospital where I used to practice. And I note that although my hospital is a little lower than some of the other hospitals in the area, it is higher than other hospitals in the State.

And as a physician, I also will submit to you that is useful information. And if recognizing the decision that a patient makes to go to a hospital is likely driven by the physician, making this type of information more available to physicians perhaps could help with physician behavior as far as directing the course for hospital care.

So, I ask unanimous consent to place this into the record, and look forward to hearing from our witnesses.

Ms. DEGETTE. Mr. Chairman, I reserve the right to object till I review the documents, although I am sure they will be fine. If I could just review the documents.

Mr. HARPER. Well, as we review that we will come back to approving the entering that into the record as soon as Ms. DeGette has had an opportunity to review that.

I will now recognize Mr. Pallone, the Ranking Member, for purposes of an opening statement.

OPENING STATEMENT OF HON. FRANK PALLONE, JR., A REPRESENTATIVE IN CONGRESS FROM THE STATE OF NEW JERSEY

Mr. PALLONE. Thank you, Mr. Chairman.

The cost of healthcare is consistently a top concern for American families. But all too often, consumers face an initial problem before they even receive care, knowing how much a certain healthcare service is going to cost them. And that is because there are so many players in the healthcare industry making it difficult to bring clear cost transparency to the consumer.

Two different patients can receive the same service from a doctor but end up being charged starkly different prices. And this makes it difficult for a patient to make an informed decision about their care.

There are multiple factors contributing to this lack of transparency in healthcare. For example, a provider may have a set of rates it changes for private-pay customers, but depending on a person's insurance and deductible, their price could vary greatly.

This differs from most other markets the consumer has a clear understanding of how much a product or service will cost, and can shop around to obtain the best deal. The nature of healthcare makes this more complicated. And it is particularly noticeable in emergency situations where a patient's top concern is receiving the lifesaving care they need, rather than what the care will cost. In other expensive specialties such as oncology, patients trust their doctors to provide them with referrals based on quality of care.

With that being said, consumers can certainly benefit from more information, and there are opportunities to bring more transparency to the healthcare industry. As we will hear from the witnesses today, just about every state has implemented some type of transparency initiative. For instance, my home State of New Jersey recently passed a law requiring providers to notify patients if they are out-of-network, helping to avoid surprise bills for patients.

Many states have also created websites that post the prices of common procedures, and allow consumers to browse the prices of various providers. And this kind of reform can empower consumers just by giving them greater access to information.

So, I look forward to hearing from the witnesses what the research says about these efforts, and what other reforms are being attempted in other states. However, we should be cautiously optimistic about greater transparency, as we have seen only modest results in actually bringing down costs. Some studies have found an increase in prices with more transparency, so we should be mindful of these results before considering any reforms.

I also think it is important that we keep the big picture in mind here. It is one thing to bring more transparency to healthcare, and give consumers information on what they are being charged, but we should also encourage meaningful efforts to actually reduce healthcare costs for American families.

And one of the primary ways to do that is by ensuring access to affordable health coverage. Whether it be Medicaid, essential health benefits in private insurance, or a robust marketplace for individuals who shop for insurance, transparency matters only if consumers have access to high-quality, affordable healthcare.

And, finally, while I appreciate the efforts of this subcommittee to explore these issues, I would be remiss if I did not note that there is an emergency taking place right now within HHS that this committee should be holding an oversight hearing on. Today, there are still more than 2,500 children in the custody of HHS who have yet to be reunited with their families after being forcibly separated by the Trump administration. This committee has a responsibility to conduct vigorous oversight of the Federal Government, and today would have been a perfect day to have HHS Secretary Azar and Scott Lloyd, the Director of the Office of Refugee Resettlement to be here.

So, I again urge the Republican majority to schedule a hearing as soon as possible so we can work to fix this crisis, and so we can finally get some answers.

I don't know if anybody wants my time. If not, I will yield back.

Thank you, Mr. Chairman.

[The prepared statement of Mr. Pallone follows:]

PREPARED STATEMENT OF HON. FRANK PALLONE, JR.

The cost of healthcare is consistently a top concern for American families. But all too often, consumers face an initial problem before they even receive care, knowing how much a certain healthcare service is going to cost them. That's because there are so many players in the healthcare industry making it difficult to bring clear cost transparency to the consumer.

Two different patients can receive the same service from a doctor but end up being charged starkly different prices. This makes it difficult for a patient to make an informed decision about their care.

There are multiple factors contributing to this lack of transparency in healthcare. For example, a provider may have a set rate it charges for private-pay customers, but depending on a person's insurance and deductible, their price could vary greatly.

This differs from most other markets, where the consumer has a clear understanding of how much a product or service will cost, and can shop around to obtain the best deal. The nature of healthcare makes this more complicated. And it's particularly noticeable in emergency situations where a patient's top concern is receiving the lifesaving care they need, rather than what that care will cost. In other expensive specialties such as oncology, patients trust their doctors to provide them with referrals based on quality of care.

That being said, consumers can certainly benefit from more information, and there are opportunities to bring more transparency to the healthcare industry. As we will hear from the witnesses today, just about every state has implemented some type of transparency initiative. For instance, my home State of New Jersey recently passed a law requiring providers to notify patients if they are out-of-network, helping to avoid surprise bills for patients.

Many states have also created websites that post the prices of common procedures, and allow consumers to browse the prices at various providers. This kind of reform can empower a consumer just by giving them greater access to information. I look forward to hearing from the witnesses what the research says about these efforts, and what other reforms are being attempted by the states. However, we should be cautiously optimistic about greater transparency, as we have seen only modest results in actually bringing down costs. Some studies have even found an increase in prices with more transparency, so we should be mindful of these results before considering any reforms.

I also think it is important that we keep the big picture in mind here. It is one thing to bring more transparency to healthcare, and give consumers information on what they are being charged, but we should also encourage meaningful efforts to actually reduce healthcare costs for American families.

And one of the primary ways to do that is by ensuring access to affordable health coverage. Whether it be Medicaid, essential health benefits in private insurance, or a robust marketplace for individuals to shop for insurance—transparency matters only if consumers have access to high-quality, affordable healthcare.

Finally, while I appreciate the efforts of this subcommittee to explore these issues, I would be remiss if I did not note that there is an emergency taking place right now within HHS that this Committee should be holding an oversight hearing on. Today, there are still more than 2,500 children in the custody of HHS who have yet to be reunited with their families after being forcibly separated by the Trump Administration. This Committee has a responsibility to conduct vigorous oversight of the Federal Government, and today would have been a perfect day to have HHS Secretary Azar and Scott Lloyd, the Director of the Office of Refugee Resettlement.

I again urge the Republican Majority to schedule a hearing as soon as possible so we can work to fix this crisis, and so we can finally get answers.

Mr. HARPER. The gentleman yields back.

Ms. DEGETTE. Mr. Chairman, I withdraw my right to object. I have no objection to these documents from Mr. Burgess.

Mr. HARPER. The documents are so entered.

[The information appears at the conclusion of the hearing.]

Mr. HARPER. I ask unanimous consent that the members' written opening, opening statements be made part of the record.

Without objection, they will be entered into the record.

Mr. HARPER. I would now like to introduce our witnesses for today.

Today we have Dr. Jaime King, Professor at UC Hastings College of Law; and Dr. Michael Chernew, Professor at the Department of Health Care Policy at Harvard Medical School.

Unfortunately, our third witness, Dr. Kavita Patel, was unable to be here today due to a family emergency. And Dr. Patel and her family will remain in our thoughts and prayers as we send them our best wishes.

You are both aware that the committee is holding an investigative hearing, and when doing so has had the practice of taking testimony under oath. Do either of you have any objection to testifying under oath?

Mr. CHERNEW. No objection. Ms. KING. No objection.

Mr. HARPER. Both witnesses have stated no.

The Chair then advises you that under the rules of the House and the rules of the committee you are entitled to be accompanied by counsel. Do you desire to be accompanied by counsel during your testimony today?

Mr. CHERNEW. No.

Ms. KING. No.

Mr. HARPER. Both witnesses have responded no.

In that case, if you would please rise and raise your right hand and I will swear you in.

[Witnesses sworn.]

Mr. HARPER. You may be seated.

You are now under oath and subject to the penalties set forth in Title 18, Section 1001, of the United States Code. You may now each give a five-minute summary of your written statement. And Dr. King, we will recognize you for 5 minutes.

Statement of Jaime King, Ph.D., Professor, UC Hastings College of Law; and Michael Chernew, Ph.D., Professor, Department of Health Care Policy, Harvard Medical School

Statement of Jaime King

Ms. KING. Thank you. Committee Chairman Walden, Subcommittee Chairman Harper, Committee Ranking Members Pallone and DeGette, Subcommittee Chairmen Griffith and Castor, and members of the Subcommittee on Oversight and Investigations, I very much appreciate the opportunity to testify on price transparency in the healthcare market today.

As you know, the cost of healthcare in the United States currently threatens the economic stability of our citizens, our businesses, and our nation. A 2018 Gallup poll found that more Americans worry about the availability and affordability of healthcare than any of the 14 other major social issues, like crime, the economy, and the availability of guns.

Economic theory suggests that if consumers had better access to price information prior to choosing providers and receiving healthcare services that they would choose less expensive options, thereby lowering overall healthcare spending. As a result, states have been very active in this endeavor, introducing 163 price transparency bills so far in 2018.

Historically, most state price transparency initiatives have focused on changing consumer behavior to encourage them to select providers and services that offer the greatest value at the lowest cost. Yet, health services research examining the impact of these efforts suggest that most of them have not engaged patients in a sufficient way to curb healthcare spending. Controlling healthcare spending requires engagement not just form patients but from all actors in the healthcare market: providers, payers, and policy makers.

Twenty states, including Oregon, Maryland, Maine, and New Hampshire, have all developed All Payer Claims Databases which collect information on both healthcare services Americans use, and amounts paid for those services. States can use these healthcare claims data to report better reporting to an All Care Claims Database, to inform patient and provider decisions regarding care; to allow payers to compare their rates to make sure that they are getting, you know, close to average or somewhere in there; and to allow policy makers to examine the drivers of healthcare costs over time; evaluate the effectiveness of various reform efforts; and measure the impact of mergers and acquisitions on healthcare price and quality.

However, legal barriers including contractual provisions, ERISA preemption, and trade secret laws currently hinder the utility of many existing price transparency initiatives.

So, what can Congress do? For transparency initiatives to achieve their full effect at the state level, changes are needed at the Federal level. And, fortunately, Congress has the ability to address some of the most significant barriers to price transparency. There are five things Congress can do to improve healthcare price transparency:

Number one, and most important, address the ERISA preemption challenges. The main goal of ERISA is to promote uniformity in state regulations governing employee benefit plans. But over time, ERISA's preemptive reach has expanded in ways that put this goal of uniformity for employers over transparency, competition, and affordability of healthcare for all Americans.

The Supreme Court decision in Gobeille v. Liberty Mutual Insurance held that ERISA preempted state All Payer Claims Databases, preempted their reporting requirements as applied to self-insured employer plans. And this decision left state All Payer Claims Databases without healthcare claims data for about a third of their population, which greatly limits their accuracy and their utility.

Essentially, trying to analyze the healthcare landscape using data from an All Payer Claims Database without the self-insured employer population is kind of akin to Google Maps, trying to use Google Maps without a third of the road; right?

Enabling All Payer Claims Databases to collect the full set of healthcare claims data would dramatically increase the utility and reliability of these initiatives. While addressing ERISA preemption of state health reform laws is the most important thing that Congress can do to promote price transparency and bring down healthcare costs, additional actions by Congress could also help illuminate healthcare prices, which brings me to number two.

Congress should seek to encourage price shopping incentives like reference pricing, rewards, and shared networks, through demonstration and pilot projects.

Number three, Congress should create a public interest exemption to Defend Trade Secrets Act of 2016. Healthcare providers and insurers currently invoke trade secrets protection to avoid disclosing negotiated healthcare prices and other information to consumer, employers, researchers, and state officials.

Trade secrets protections were designed to encourage and protect innovation, like the Coca-Cola formula, not to permit Coca-Cola and restauranteurs to hide its price on the menu and then after you eat your meal give you a bill for a $25 Coke. Right?

Number four, Congress should require manufacturers of electronic medical records and insurance companies to establish uniform standards of interoperability and standard bundles of care for billing purposes so that providers and patients can access meaningful and actionable information about the cost to the patient, who and what is in the patient's network, and the quality of providers and services being offered to them when the provider is making referrals during appointments.

And, number five, they should develop billing codes for a physician's time spent in these efforts.

Thank you.

[The prepared statement of Ms. King follows:]

TESTIMONY OF: JAIME S. KING, EXAMINING STATE EFFORTS TO IMPROVE TRANSPARENCY IN HEALTHCARE COSTS FOR CONSUMERS, SUBCOMMITTEE ON OVERSIGHT AND INVESTIGATIONS COMMITTEE ON ENERGY AND COMMERCE, U.S. HOUSE OF REPRESENTATIVES, TUESDAY, JULY 17, 2018

Summary of Testimony

The United States currently spends more than any other nation on healthcare, as a percentage of gross domestic product and per capita. Our healthcare markets suffer from high levels of consolidation, a lack of clear price and quality signals for consumers, and an inability to access price, utilization, and quality data. Price transparency initiatives, like all payer claims databases, can improve healthcare market functioning in all these areas by providing relevant information to decision-makers, including patients, providers, payers, and policymakers, at key decision points. Historically, most price transparency initiatives have focused on changing consumer behavior to encourage them to select providers and services that provide the greatest value at the lowest cost. Unfortunately, these initiatives have not been successful at bending the cost curve due to limited usage and mixed levels of effectiveness. Price transparency initiatives that provide patient, provider, procedure, and plan level of specificity on price and quality to consumers, accompanied by a financial incentive, like reference pricing or tiering, have proven more effective. However, even with these potential improvements, legal barriers including contractual provisions, ERISA preemption, and trade secrets laws continue to hinder the utility of many existing price transparency initiatives.

Congress, more than any other entity, has the ability to address the most significant barriers to price transparency in healthcare and maximize the tremendous untapped potential of existing state initiatives, in particular APCDs. To do so, Congress should narrow ERISA preemption to exclude state health reform efforts that do not unduly burden ERISA's goal of uniformity for employer-based benefit plans, while also granting states sufficient flexibility to achieve their health reform goals.

Testimony of Jaime S. King

Committee Chairman Walden, Subcommittee Chairman Harper, Committee Ranking Member Pallone, Subcommittee Ranking Member Degette, and Members of the Subcommittee on Oversight and Investigations, I very much appreciate the opportunity to testify on the role of price transparency in the healthcare market. I am a professor of law and the Bion M. Gregory Chair in Business Law at the University of California, Hastings College of the Law. I have written and taught in the field of health law and policy for the last ten years. I am also the Associate Dean and Co-Director of the UCSF/UC Hastings Consortium on Law, Science and Health Policy, and the Co-Founder and Executive Editor of The Source on Healthcare Price and Competition, a free and independent academic website that posts news, academic articles, legislative developments, litigation documents, original analysis, and guest commentary on healthcare price and competition. I owe a great deal of thanks to Katherine Gudiksen, Laura Hagen, Erin Fuse Brown, Anna Sinaiko, and everyone at The Source on Healthcare Price and Competition who contributed their time, effort, and research to this testimony.

Introduction

The cost of healthcare in the United States currently threatens the economic stability of our citizens, our businesses, our state and local governments, and our nation. The United States spends more on healthcare than on any other sector of the economy, including defense, transportation, education, or housing. A 2018 Gallup poll found that a greater percentage of Americans (55%) stated that they worry "a great deal" about the availability and affordability of healthcare than fourteen other major social issues, like crime, the economy, unemployment, terrorist attacks, and the availability of guns.[1] In 2017, projected U.S. spending on healthcare goods and services approached $3.5 trillion.[2] This amounts to more than any other economically developed country, both as a percentage of GDP and per capita.[3] Despite this, the health of Americans is not significantly better than that of our counterparts in countries like the U.K. or Canada. In fact, on many key metrics we are falling behind.[4]

When faced with how to address growing healthcare costs, academics and policymakers frequently focus on ways to address market inefficiencies and failures. One market failure that has received a great deal of attention in recent years is the lack of price transparency in the healthcare market. Nearly every day a news story reveals the plight of Americans facing astronomical healthcare bills that seem to have little to no relation to the cost of providing the services received and come as a complete shock to consumers. For instance, Peter Drier of New York was blindsided by a medical bill of about $117,000 from an "assistant surgeon" who the primary surgeon called in while Mr. Drier was receiving neck surgery. Each surgeon billed for each step of the procedure. The primary surgeon billed $74,000 for removing two disks and an additional $50,000 for placing the hardware, while the assistant billed $67,000 and $50,000 for those tasks. The primary surgeon accepted a negotiated fee determined through Mr. Drier's insurance company which was about $6,200. However, because the assistant surgeon was out-of-network, he charged

---

[1] Jeffrey Jones, *U.S. Concerns About Healthcare High; Energy, Unemployment Low*, GALLUP (March 26, 2018), https://news.gallup.com/poll/231533/concerns-healthcare-high-energy-unemployment-low.aspx.

[2] CENTERS FOR MEDICARE AND MEDICAID SERVICES, NATIONAL HEALTH EXPENDITURES FACT SHEET, https://www.cms.gov/research-statistics-data-and-systems/statistics-trends-and-reports/nationalhealthexpenddata/nhe-fact-sheet.html (last modified Apr. 17, 2018).

[3] ORGANIZATION FOR ECONOMIC COOPERATION AND DEVELOPMENT, SPENDING ON HEALTH: LATEST TRENDS, June 2018, http://www.oecd.org/health/health-systems/health-data.htm.

[4] Irene Papanicolas et al., *Health Care Spending in the United States and Other High-Income Countries*, 319 JAMA 10, 1024-39 (2018); Austin Frakt, *Medical Mystery: Something Happened to U.S. Health Spending After 1980*, N.Y. TIMES (May 14, 2018), https://www.nytimes.com/2018/05/14/upshot/medical-mystery-health-spending-1980.html.

$117,000. Had Mr. Drier been a Medicare beneficiary, the assistant would have only been able to bill 16% of the primary surgeon's fee – roughly $800, less than 1% of what the assistant surgeon was actually paid.[5] In an effort to protect patients like Mr. Drier from these astronomical fees, and twenty-four states enacted legislation prohibiting surprise billing of patients.[6]

Economic theory suggests that if consumers had better access to price information prior to choosing providers and receiving healthcare services, they would choose less expensive providers and services, and thereby lower overall healthcare spending. Empirical studies on price transparency in other markets show that transparency initiatives tend to lead to more consistent, lower prices.[7] As a result, price transparency has become a "cornerstone of the consumer-directed healthcare model," with policymakers, insurers, private entities, state and local governments, and consumer advocacy organizations investing significant time, resources, and capital to promote consumer-focused price transparency in healthcare.[8] Yet, health services research examining the impact of these efforts suggests that most of them have not engaged patients in a sufficient way to curb healthcare spending.[9]

---

[5] Elisabeth Rosenthal, *After Surgery, Surprise $117,000 Medical Bill from Doctor He Didn't Know*, N.Y. TIMES (Sept. 14, 2014), https://www.nytimes.com/2014/09/21/us/drive-by-doctoring-surprise-medical-bills.html.

[6] *See* Kevin Lucia et al., *Balance Billing by Health Care Providers: Assessing Consumer Protections Across States*, THE COMMONWEALTH FUND (June 13, 2017), https://www.commonwealthfund.org/publications/issue-briefs/2017/jun/balance-billing-health-care-providers-assessing-consumer for a description of 21 states that had balance billing laws in 2017. Since the report was issued, Tennessee (HB 1935/SB 1969), Minnesota (SF 3480), and Missouri (SB 982) have passed balanced billing laws and Colorado (SB 146/HB 1282), New Hampshire (HB 1782/HB 1809), and New Jersey (AB 2039) have strengthened theirs.

[7] D. ANDREW AUSTIN & JANE G. GRAVELLE, CRS Report for Congress: Does Price Transparency Effect Market Efficiency? Implications of Empirical Evidence in Other Markets for the Healthcare Sector (2008) [hereinafter CRS Report for Congress].

[8] A. Mehrotra et al., *Promise and Reality of Price Transparency*, 378 N. ENGL. J. MED. 14, 1348 (2018).

[9] *See, e.g.*, A. Mehrotra et al., *Use Patterns of a State Health Care Price Transparency Web Site: What Do Patients Shop For?*, 51 INQUIRY: THE J. OF HEALTH CARE ORG., PROVISION, AND FINANCING, 0046958014561496 (2014); S. Desai et al., *Association Between Availability of a Price Transparency Tool and Outpatient Spending*, 315 JAMA 17, 1874-81 (2016).

Controlling healthcare spending requires engagement from all stakeholders in the healthcare market – patients, providers, payers, and policymakers. Price transparency initiatives, such as all payer claims databases (APCDs), have great potential to provide critical data to guide healthcare reform efforts, inform analysis on the drivers of healthcare costs, and help patients and providers choose high-value/lower-cost treatment options. However, currently the amount and quality of data available to patients and their doctors and laws restricting data collection limit even premier price transparency tools.

My testimony today will provide an overview of existing price transparency tools, and then focus on how improved transparency can benefit healthcare decision-making by targeting different information to stakeholders. I will then discuss why many prior attempts at improving price transparency have not achieved their goals, and what Congress can do to promote price transparency in healthcare.

Summary of Key Points

- Price transparency initiatives can improve healthcare market functioning by providing relevant information to decision-makers, including consumers, providers, insurers, employers, and policymakers, at key decision points.
- Historically, most price transparency initiatives have focused on changing consumer behavior to encourage them to select lower priced providers and services. These initiatives have had limited usage and mixed results.
- Price transparency initiatives that provide patient, provider, procedure, and plan level of specificity on price and quality to consumers, accompanied by a financial incentive, like reference pricing or tiering, have proven more effective.
- Legal barriers including contractual provisions, ERISA preemption, and trade secrets laws hinder the effectiveness of many existing price transparency initiatives.

- Congress has a range of options in how it can promote price transparency to improve healthcare decision-making and lower costs, but the most important and effective act it could take is to leverage existing state efforts and resources by amending ERISA to narrow its preemption of state health reform efforts, especially those targeting transparency.

Overview of State Price Transparency Initiatives

Over the last ten years, states have passed laws to reduce the barriers to price transparency and developed statewide databases of healthcare claims data to allow for comparison and analysis of healthcare price, quality, and utilization data. State governments have refined their transparency tools over time to improve their utility and to respond to particularly pressing issues. So far in 2018, state legislatures have introduced 163 healthcare price transparency bills (see Appendix A). A large percentage of these bills focused on addressing transparency in pharmaceutical drug prices, but states have also introduced a wide swath of non-pharmaceutical price transparency bills. Recent state-based efforts include implementing and expanding APCDs, giving consumers new tools to access and compare prices for both insurance plans and healthcare services, and incentivizing patients to shop for higher-value services. Finally, many states recently passed laws protecting patients from surprise or balance billing practices, and laws prohibiting anti-competitive contract terms like gag clauses and anti-tiering/anti-steering clauses. This section will highlight some of the most common state transparency initiatives.

All Payer Claims Databases

All Payer Claims Databases (APCDs) are the cornerstone of many comprehensive price transparency initiatives. Their importance to developing consumer shopping tools, public informational tools, healthcare cost control efforts, and overall competition in healthcare markets cannot be overstated. An APCD is a comprehensive collection of medical claims data from both public and private payers with information specific to individual plans, patients, and procedures. Consumers can use the data in APCDs to shop for higher value health services or providers. In addition, data from APCDs can be used to inform state policymakers about the operation of healthcare markets in the state.

While APCDs are instrumental tools for consumer shopping, they typically collect information on the services provided and the *amounts paid* for those services, rather than the *fees charged.* Insurance companies negotiate significant discounts from retail or "chargemaster" rates, and so such rates rarely provide the critical pricing information that patients and policymakers need. Providing both negotiated prices and amounts paid, on the other hand, paints a much clearer picture, though they are notoriously difficult to access.

To obtain such information, many states have mandated health plans to report their prices to the state APCD, while others permit them to submit the information voluntarily. Maine established the first statewide APCD in 2003, and twenty states now have or are implementing statewide APCDs with mandatory submission, and seven more states have APCDs, with voluntary submission.[10] States with mandatory reporting requirements have more comprehensive data. States with only voluntary reporting mechanisms only receive a portion of the picture, which will, almost assuredly, not prove representative of the entire population. For example, Oklahoma's voluntary APCD covers only 1 million people, or approximately 25% of the population,[11] and therefore risks giving misleading information.

The demand for more reliable information about costs is growing and experts predict that over half the states will have an APCD or APCD-like database by 2022 that will cover at least two-thirds of their populations.[12] States will continue to improve and refine their APCDs. However, the

[10] The states with APCDs that require submission are: AR, CO, CT, DE, FL, HI, KS, ME, MD, MA, MN, NH, NY, OR, RI, TN, UT, VT, WA, WV. The states with voluntary APCDs are: CA, MI, OK, SC, VA, WI, WY. https://www.apcdcouncil.org/.

[11] *Oklahoma*, APCD COUNCIL, https://www.apcdcouncil.org/ (last visited July 11, 2018).

[12] Joel Ario & Kevin McAvey, *Transparency in Health Care: Where We Stand And What Policy Makers Can Do Now*, HEALTH AFFAIRS BLOG (July 11, 2018), https://www.healthaffairs.org/do/10.1377/hblog20180703.549221/full/.

reliability and utility of state APCDs are compromised by their inability to obtain a comprehensive set of claims data because ERISA preempts any state law requiring self-insured employers to submit healthcare claims data. Nonetheless, the experience of many states demonstrates the power of APCDs to both help patients shop for higher value care and strengthen analysis of a state's healthcare market.

Price Comparison Tools

Once established, states can use the data collected in their APCD to create price comparison tools and incentives for patients to find the best value providers. For example, NH Health Cost, New Hampshire's APCD-based consumer-facing website, allows consumers, health plan enrollees, and employers to select different carriers while comparing prices.[13] Importantly, because NH Health Cost has access to the insurer's negotiated prices with in-network providers, it can provide consumers with personalized out-of-pocket cost information for a particular procedure with a particular provider. New Hampshire's website is also one of the few publicly available sites that allows employers or payers to compare their rates to the median rate for a given service at a particular provider (e.g., a colonoscopy at the same hospital for each major insurer). Even with the desire and expertise, New Hampshire has struggled to offer this level of detailed information for each patient as benefit designs evolve to include options like value-based payments.[14]

Massachusetts, another pioneer in building and refining APCDs, also requires mandatory submission of healthcare claims data and records of services provided from public and private payers, including commercial health plans, Medicare, and MassHealth.[15] However, Massachusetts' APCD, maintained by the Center for Health Information and Analysis (CHIA),[16] does not offer the same connectivity with specific insurance

---

[13] NH HEALTH COST, https://nhhealthcost.nh.gov/ (last visited July 11, 2018).
[14] Ario & McAvey, *supra* note 13.
[15] In Massachusetts, Medicaid and Children's Health Insurance Program (CHIP) are combined into one program called MassHealth. *MassHealth*, MASS.GOV, https://www.mass.gov/topics/masshealth (last visited July 11, 2018).
[16] CHIA, http://www.chiamass.gov/ (last visited July 11, 2018).

plans as New Hampshire's APCD does. Instead, CHIA's healthcare transparency tool, MassCompareCare, includes a procedure pricing tool. This tool uses data extracted from the state's 2015 APCD and displays, by insurer, the median payment to any provider for any of 295 services. Additionally, it supplies quality information about different providers.

While these consumer-facing websites offer patients pricing information for different providers and services, few patients have engaged with them, for reasons I discuss below, and states have begun to try to incentivize patient engagement.

Right to Shop Laws

"Right to Shop" laws attempt to engage patients by giving them the ability to benefit financially when they choose lower-cost care. In New Hampshire, for example, consumers who successfully select a provider/service at a lower price receive a share of the savings in cash.[17] Maine adopted a similar Right to Shop law in 2017 with transparency provisions that require insurers to give patients access to anticipated charges and estimated out-of-pocket charges in advance of receiving care. The law also requires carriers with small business group plans to offer plans that give financial incentives to patients who choose a high-quality, low-cost provider, and to require all non-HMO plans to cover out-of-network providers with rates that are lower than the state average.[18] In order to implement Right to Shop laws, states and/or providers must first build comprehensive databases, such as APCDs, and implement shopping tools necessary to allow consumers to accurately and adequately shop between providers and services.

Restrictions on Surprise and/or Balance Billing

Other efforts to improve price transparency focus on providing patients access to prices when they seek care and protecting them from surprise

---

[17] N.H. REV. STAT. ANN. § 420-G:11, G:11-a (2018); Josh Archambault & Nic Horton, *Right to Shop: The Next Big Thing in Health Care*, FORBES (Aug. 5, 2016, 12:12 PM), https://www.forbes.com/sites/theapothecary/2016/08/05/right-to-shop-the-next-big-thing-in-health-care.

[18] L.D. 445, 128th Leg., Reg. Sess. (Me. 2018).

bills. When an insured patient sees an out-of-network provider, the provider can bill the patient for the difference between the provider's charges and the insurer's payment. These surprise or balance billing practices can result in astronomical out-of-pocket costs for patients, as Peter Drier of New York found out when he got the bill for $117,000 from the assistant surgeon that he never met. These practices often affect patients in their weakest moments when they have little control over their care (e.g., in a hospital where they receive care from an out-of-network doctor at an in-network facility). In response, states have begun taking action to restrict surprise and balance billing.

Currently 24 states offer some protection from balance billing, but only less than half offer comprehensive safeguards.[19] While some states, including Florida,[20] California,[21] and, more recently, New Jersey,[22] ban balance billing altogether, many states instead require some form of disclosure of potential balance or surprise billing. States have done this in different ways. For example, some states require providers to disclose that a patient might receive a bill for charges from out-of-network providers or that certain types of providers are not employed by the facility. For example, Tennessee requires health facilities to have patients sign the following statement before receiving care: "Anesthesiologists, radiologists, emergency room physicians, and pathologists are not employed by this facility... Before receiving services, the patient should check with his or her insurance carrier to find out if the patient's providers are in-network.

Otherwise, the patient may be at risk of higher out-of-network charges."[23] These type of disclosure laws, however, do little more than

[19] See footnote 6. According to Lucia 2017, some states prohibit provider balance billing, while others require insurers to hold enrollees harmless from balance billing charges by paying the entire charge if necessary, and some do both. In states that have adopted both approaches, out-of-network providers are directly prohibited from balance billing consumers for additional charges beyond what the health plan pays. In addition, insurers must guarantee that the consumer is held harmless from, and is not liable for, balance billing charges.

[20] H.B. 221, Reg. Sess. (Fla. 2016).

[21] A.B. 72, Reg. Sess. (Cal. 2018).

[22] A.B. 2039, Reg. Sess. (N.J. 2018).

[23] H.B. 1935 & S.B. 1869, 110th Leg., Reg. Sess. (Tenn. 2018) (codified at TENN. CODE ANN. § 56-7-120 (2018)) requires written consent for both the charges and the out-of-network statement.

cover the providers from liability, as patients often have little choice of emergency room physician or anesthesiologist. Without adequate information and viable options, patients have little ability to plan for or avoid such costs. The goal of price transparency initiatives is to reduce expenditures by allowing patients to shop for higher value care. Patients will be unable to meaningfully shop for care if they cannot know the prices before getting that care, they do not have a choice in providers, or if they may be charged excessively high fees that they could not anticipate.

Some states require disclosure of cost estimates. Minnesota requires providers to give patients good faith estimates of the payment the provider has agreed to accept from the consumer's health plan and to disclose any fees, including facility fees, that an insurer does not typically pay.[24] Some states have gone a bit further and passed "hold harmless laws." For example, Colorado requires a provider to accept payment that is equal to the rate the insurer would pay to an in-network provider.[25] Colorado, however, does not prohibit providers from sending bills to patients who might not understand that they do not have a responsibility to pay those bills.[26] By prohibiting surprise billing practices and requiring providers and insurers to negotiate out-of-network rates, at least for emergency services, states can protect patients from financially devastating and unavoidable healthcare bills.

Prohibitions on Anti-Transparency Contract Provisions

States have also begun to prohibit insurers and providers from including certain types of provisions in their contracts that might prevent disclosure of healthcare prices or price shopping. First, non-disclosure provisions, also known as "gag clauses," often prohibit providers and insurers from disclosing negotiated prices, methods of cost-sharing, or more affordable treatment options. In 2017, Maine passed a law

---

[24] Minnesota Senate Bill 3480, which recently passed, requires provider to provide the consumer with information regarding other types of fees or charges that the consumer may be required to pay in conjunction with a visit to the provider, including but not limited to any applicable facility fees. S.F. 3480, 90th Leg., Reg. Sess. (Minn. 2018).

[25] S.B. 06-213, 65th Leg., 2nd Reg. Sess. (Colo.2006).

[26] Lucia, *supra* note 6.

prohibiting gag clauses in pharmacy contracts, which states "if information related to an enrollee's out-of-pocket cost or the clinical efficacy of a prescription drug or alternative medication is available to a pharmacy provider, a carrier or pharmacy benefits manager may not penalize a pharmacy provider for providing that information to an enrollee."[27] In other instances, higher-priced providers have used anti-tiering or anti-steering contract provisions to prevent insurers from incentivizing patients to choose lower-cost providers. For example, insurers could signal which providers offer higher value care through the use of "tiered networks" by offering lower copays or other cost-sharing reductions to patients who use providers in preferred tiers. Most famously, North Carolina and the Department of Justice recently sued the Carolinas HealthCare System in an antitrust suit, claiming that the provider's anti-tiering and anti-steering provisions violated Section 1 of the Sherman Act.[28] California is currently considering a bill to ban these contract provisions, but it has not yet passed.[29]

Naming and Shaming Laws

In contrast to transparency laws that encourage or enable patients to make more cost-effective decisions about healthcare, laws that publicly display and/or fine entities with high healthcare prices aim to alert the public as to which entities are charging the highest prices and potentially shame them into lowering prices. In "naming and shaming laws," states may also explicitly define price gouging, often saying if prices increase higher than some threshold without a reasonable justification, the state Attorney General can prosecute the entity for price gouging. In 2018, most naming and shaming laws focused on addressing drug prices; however, states could apply similar laws to non-pharmaceutical healthcare services in the future.

---

[27] L.D. 6, 128th Leg., Reg. Sess. (Me. 2017) (codified at ME. REV. STAT. ANN. tit. 24-a, § 4317 (2018)).

[28] *United States and the State of North Carolina v. The Charlotte-Mecklenburg Hosp. Auth., d/b/a Carolinas Healthcare System*, 248 F. Supp. 3d 720 (W.D.N.C. 2017). *See also United States v. Am. Express Co.*, 838 F.3d 179 (2d Cir. 2016).

[29] S.B. 538, Reg. Sess. (Cal. 2018).

The states have demonstrated a keen interest in addressing healthcare costs and promoting healthcare price transparency. State laws have evolved over time to better satisfy consumer and governmental needs to access healthcare pricing data, yet there is still a long way to go.

The Unrealized Potential of Consumer-Focused Transparency Tools

With all the interest in state price transparency initiatives, one would think they had been quite successful at lowering healthcare spending. Despite growing efforts at both the state and federal level to increase transparency as a means of facilitating price shopping, so far these tools have been ineffective at substantially reducing costs. Studies examining these tools repeatedly demonstrate that simply offering patients access to price transparency tools alone has little effect on healthcare spending.[30,31,32]

Initially, price transparency tools offered patients provider retail rates, known as "chargemaster" rates. These provide little utility for insured patients attempting to know their out-of-pocket costs for a particular procedure by a particular provider within their particular plan. Patients also found the information on these websites confusing, as the terms and procedures were not standardized, the billing mechanisms were highly complex, and the prices often were broken out across a range of providers, services, and devices, making it impossible for a patient to fully anticipate his or her costs. Not surprisingly, consumers did not use these tools very often.

Over time, states and insurers offering consumer-facing price comparison tools, like NH Health Costs or United Healthcare's MyUHC

---

[30] Ethan M.J. Lieber, *Does It Pay to Know Prices in Health Care?*, 9 AM. ECON. J.: ECON. POL'Y 1, 154-79 (2017).

[31] Sunita Desai et al., *Offering a Price Transparency Tool Did Not Reduce Overall Spending Among California Public Employees and Retirees*, 36 HEALTH AFFAIRS 8, 1401-7 (2017).

[32] Anna D. Sinaiko et al., *Association Between Viewing Health Care Price Information and Choice of Health Care Facility*, 176 *JAMA Internal Medicine* 12, 1868-70 (2016).

Cost Estimator,[33] began to offer consumers information on their out-of-pocket prices that that were patient, provider, procedure, and plan specific. For a price transparency tool to be useful for consumers, it must tell them how different choices of providers will affect *their* costs. When a patient uses a price transparency tool, studies have typically found savings between 10 and 17% for that patient.[34,35] These results are promising, but research demonstrates that the effect on overall spending is minimal due to lack of consumer engagement with these tools.

Overwhelmingly, studies reveal patients' reluctance to use price transparency tools when shopping for medical procedures, with approximately 2-20% of patients using available tools to search for price information, depending on the intervention.[36,37,38,39,40] For example, in a 2016 study, only 3.5% of Aetna enrollees used an available online, personalized, episode-level price comparison tool, but costs for enrollees that used the tool to search for diagnostic services were 12% less than those who did not use the tool.[41] Further, a study by Desai et al. showed that access to a price transparency website led to only a 1% decrease in medical spending because less than 10% of eligible patients even logged into the online tool to search for any procedure or provider.[42] Mehotra et al. attempted to understand how patients seek out price information by interviewing 3,000 non-elderly Americans with recent out-of-pocket spending on medical services.[43] The researchers found that 13% of the interviewees had searched for price information before their care, but in

---

[33] *MyUHC Cost Estimator*, UNITED HEALTHCARE, https://www.uhc.com/individual-and-family/member-resources/health-care-tools/cost-estimator. (last visited July 14, 2018).

[34] Lieber, *supra* note 31.

[35] C. Whaley et al., *Association Between Availability of Health Service Prices and Payments for these Services*, 312 *JAMA* 16, 1679-76 (2014).

[36] Lieber, *supra* note 31.

[37] Whaley et al., *supra* note 36, at 1670-76.

[38] Anna D. Sinaiko & Meredith B. Rosenthal, *Examining a Healthcare Price Transparency Tool: Who Uses It, and How They Shop for Care*, 35 HEALTH AFFAIRS 4, 662-70 (2016).

[39] Desai et al., *supra* note 32.

[40] A. Mehrotra et al., *Americans Support Price Shopping for Health Care, but Few Actually Seek Out Price Information*, 36 HEALTH AFFAIRS 8, 1392-400 (2017).

[41] Sinaiko et al., *supra* note 33.

[42] Desai et al., *supra* note 10.

[43] Mehrotra et al., *supra* note 41.

most cases the patients had only called their physician or plan to determine their out-of-pocket costs, rather than use the online tool to compare prices and select a provider. Specifically, only 3% of the interviewed patients compared prices between different providers. Because so few patients use these tools, consumer-focused price transparency tools, even those that can provide provider specific and plan specific information, have generally demonstrated minimal savings.[44]

The question is: why aren't these tools more widely used? First, most insurance benefit designs do not incentivize patients to shop for costs. For example, if a patient has a flat copay, she has little financial incentive to search for a cheaper provider.[45] Second, decisions about medical care are critically important and patients are often forced to make these decisions at particularly vulnerable and challenging times. Patients often simply do not have the stamina and energy to track down different provider prices, identify those with the lowest cost rates, make numerous phone calls to see which ones are actually taking patients and still remain in their network, and then wait for their appointment. They would much prefer to receive a short list of providers recommended by their primary care doctor or loved one and seek treatment from them. Finally, since patients have so much at stake, price is often not the determining factor when making medical decisions. For shoppable services, i.e., non-urgent and interchangeable services like laboratory or diagnostic tests, patients are more willing to shop based on price, but patients are much less likely to do so for services where the quality is harder to assess, like provider selection. Detailed interviews with patients with access to the Castlight price transparency tool[46] highlighted that factors other than price are most important when choosing a provider; patients described how their relationship, trust, and loyalty to their current providers was more important than cost.[47] Patients also face significant switching costs associated with becoming a patient at a new practice, including long wait times for appointments, additional

---

[44] Mehrotra et al., *supra* note 9, at 1348-54.
[45] Lieber, *supra* note 31.
[46] CASTLIGHT HEALTH, https://www.castlighthealth.com/ (last visited July 14, 2018).
[47] H.L. Semigran et al., *Patients' Views on Price Shopping and Price Transparency*, 23 AM. J. OF MANAGED CARE 6, e186-92 (2017).

paperwork, having to recount their medical history, and loss of provider knowledge about the patient's personal and medical history. As a result, the most opportune time to offer information about costs and value to patients is when they choose new insurance coverage or new providers.

All these factors mean that healthcare services differ substantially from most other items individuals purchase. Choosing to compare prices and change providers is not like choosing to shop at a different car dealership or department store. The consequences of choosing a lower quality provider can be catastrophic and patients are often hesitant to shop for a better price, especially when making these choices without guidance and support. Furthermore, the lasting relationship patients often have with their primary care provider builds trust, and if their provider refers them to a particular specialist, patients often choose to see that particular provider without considering cost. Even individuals with high-deductible health plans (HDHPs), who seemingly have the highest financial incentives to shop for higher-value, lower-cost services, rarely switch providers or seek out lower-cost services. A study of people in the first two years of coverage under an HDHP found a 15% reduction on spending for healthcare services for these individuals.[48] Detailed economic analysis, however, showed that nearly all the savings came from reducing the amount of care the individuals received, not from price shopping or switching providers.[49]

Collectively, these studies provide evidence that, when used effectively, price transparency tools can reduce the cost of health services. These studies also show, however, that to broaden the use and impact of these tools, we need to do more than simply provide patients with access to lists of providers and prices. We must engage other actors in healthcare markets by providing them access to relevant healthcare pricing information at critical decision-making points.

---

[48] Zarek C. Brot-Goldberg et al., *What does a Deductible Do? The Impact of Cost-Sharing on Health Care Prices, Quantities, and Spending Dynamics*, 132 THE Q. J. OF ECONS. 3, 1261-1318 (2017).

[49] *Id.*

Maximizing the Potential of Price Transparency Tools

The current lack of price transparency in healthcare not only confounds patient decision-making, it also hinders provider treatment decisions, payer price setting, and governmental reform efforts and policy analysis. This section provides suggestions for how various price transparency initiatives can promote more cost effective decision-making and help bend the cost curve by providing patients, providers, payers, and policymakers essential information at critical decision points.

Patients

To maximize the effectiveness of consumer-facing price transparency tools, patients need actionable information from trusted sources and incentives to act on that information. For example, a study by Wu et al. demonstrated that when a representative of their insurer called patients, informed them about a lower-cost location for their MRI, and, if desired, helped reschedule their appointment at a high-value provider, the average cost for an MRIs decreased by 18.7% as patients shifted away from more expensive hospital-based facilities.[50] Furthermore, the authors found that prices at hospital-based facilities dropped over 10% and price variation in the metropolitan regions studied decreased by 30%, indicating that price transparency also encouraged providers to lower their price to remain competitive.[51] Perhaps most encouragingly, the authors found that all patients in these areas experienced the benefits of lowered prices through competition.[52] Entire communities benefit when the market encourages high-cost providers to lower their prices or justify higher prices with higher quality for their services.

Reference pricing provides another means of encouraging patients to use price transparency tools. When using reference pricing, an employer or insurer pays up to an established maximum price, the reference price, for a

---

[50] S.J. Wu et al., *Price Transparency for MRIs Increased Use of Less Costly Providers and Triggered Provider Competition*, 33 HEALTH AFFAIRS 8, 1391-98 (2015).

[51] *Id.* The intervention was implemented in Atlanta, GA; Cincinnati, OH; Cleveland, OH; Indianapolis, IN; and St. Louis, MO.

[52] *Id.*

healthcare service. The reference price is typically set at a level that allows patients to receive a healthcare service from multiple high-quality providers without additional contribution. The patient must pay for any costs of the service above that price, so reference pricing encourages patients to be more engaged consumers. For instance, if the reference price for an office visit to a provider is $200, the patient will receive full coverage for providers that charge $200 or less, but they will need to pay $50 extra for a provider that charges $250. Unlike HDHPs, where patients might be forced to forgo care if they cannot afford the procedure, reference pricing lowers costs while ensuring that patients can access care from a range of covered providers.

Reference pricing thus preserves a patient's ability to choose higher-priced providers if she values their services enough to pay the higher rate, and simultaneously encourages providers to drop their price to the reference price. A study by Robinson and Brown found that price transparency tools coupled with reference pricing effectively directed patients seeking orthopedic surgery to lower-cost providers and, similarly to the study by Wu et al., the costs of the procedure at high-priced facilities decreased by 30% due to price competition.[53] Studies of two of the leaders in adopting reference pricing, the California Public Employees' Retirement System (CalPERS) and the grocery firm Safeway, demonstrate the potential of coupling reference pricing and consumer price shopping. These organizations reduced spending by 20% for joint replacement,[54] 18% for cataract removal,[55] 21% for colonoscopy,[56] 17% for arthroscopy,[57]

---

[53] J.C. Robinson & T.T. Brown. *Increases in Consumer Cost Sharing Redirect Patient Volumes and Reduce Hospital Prices for Orthopedic Surgery*. 33 HEALTH AFFAIRS 8, 1392–97 (2013).

[54] *Id.*

[55] J.C. Robinson et al., *Reference-Based Benefit Design Changes Consumers' Choices and Employers' Payments for Ambulatory Surgery*, 34 HEALTH AFFAIRS, 415-22 (2015).

[56] J.C. Robinson et al., *Association of Reference Payment for Colonoscopy with Consumer Choices, Insurer Spending, and Procedural Complications*. 175 JAMA INTERNAL MEDICINE, 1783-89 (2015).

[57] J.C. Robinson et al., *Consumer Choice Between Hospital-Based and Freestanding Facilities for Arthroscopy: Impact on Prices, Spending, and Surgical Complications*. 97 THE J. OF BONE AND JOINT SURGERY, 1473-81 (2015).

12% for computed tomography,[58] and 32% for laboratory assays[59] using reference pricing. Montana also used reference pricing to control healthcare costs for beneficiaries in the state employees' health plan[60] and agreed to pay an average of 234% of Medicare rates for hospital services.[61] Since the program started in July 2016, the state has saved $15.6 million[62] and will save an estimated $25 million by the end of 2018.[63] A study by researchers at the University of California, Berkeley, estimated that if the insurers Aetna, United Healthcare, and Humana all implemented reference pricing for laboratory testing services for their commercially insured patients, collectively they would save $7.6 billion annually, or about 8% of the total spending for this population.[64]

Taken together, these studies demonstrate the potential of price transparency tools when coupled with other mechanisms to encourage their use. They further demonstrate the potential of price transparency between providers to leverage competitive forces to drive down prices. An important caveat, however, is that these studies focus on "shoppable" medical services, ones that are generally standardized and relatively interchangeable, like laboratory tests and generic drugs. In other words, they are not relationship-based services; they do not require patients to switch providers.

To bend the cost curve, however, patients need to choose lower-priced providers. As noted above, consumers have been more reluctant to use

---

[58] J.C. Robinson et al., *Reference Pricing, Consumer Cost-Sharing, and Insurer Spending for Advanced Imaging Tests*, 54 MEDICAL CARE, 1050-1055 (2016).

[59] J.C. Robinson et al., *Association of Reference Pricing for Diagnostic Laboratory Testing with Changes in Patient Choices, Prices, and Total Spending for Diagnostic Tests*, 176 JAMA INTERNAL MEDICINE, 1353-59 (2016).

[60] Julie Appleby, *Holy Cow' Moment Changes How Montana's State Health Plan Does Business*, THE WASHINGTON POST (June 20, 2018), https://www.washingtonpost.com/national/health-science/holy-cow-moment-changes-how-montanas-state-health-plan-does-business/2018/06/20/92b3693c-746a-11e8-bda1-18e53a448a14_story.html?utm_term=.df1a721650a1.

[61] Appleby, *supra* note 60.

[62] *Id.*

[63] Press Release, State of Montana Government, Governor Bullock Announces State Health Plan Change Will Save Taxpayers More Than $25 Million By End of 2018 (July 8, 2016), https://news.mt.gov/governor-bullock-announces-state-health-plan-change-will-save-taxpayers-more-than-25-million-by-end-of-2018.

[64] J.C. Robinson et al., *Reference Pricing Changes the 'Choice Architecture' of Health Care for Consumers*, 3 HEALTH AFFAIRS, 524-30 (2017).

price transparency tools to select providers. Trust and relationships are paramount for most patients, especially sick ones. A survey of people with HDHP insurance coverage showed that, while the majority of these enrollees believed there were large differences in price between providers, and that higher-cost providers were not necessarily of higher quality, they were no more likely than enrollees in traditional plans to considering switching providers or to compare out of pocket costs for a new provider.[65] Simply put, patients are reluctant to switch providers, even when it might mean substantial out-of-pocket savings.

Furthermore, the burden of lowering healthcare costs should not be placed solely on the weakest and most vulnerable link in the healthcare chain, patients. Those who can most benefit from price transparency tools are often too sick and overwhelmed to appropriately advocate for themselves and navigate the complicated labyrinth of insurance networks, plan benefit design, and healthcare prices. The stakes are simply too high for individuals – one misstep could result in financial ruin, loss of a home, or bankruptcy. Other actors in the healthcare market, including providers, employers, insurers, and policymakers, should also leverage price transparency tools to lower costs.

Providers

Primary care providers are uniquely well-positioned to use price transparency tools to guide patients toward lower-cost providers when making decisions about which specialist to see and which treatment options to consider. Patients often want an informed referral or recommendation from a trusted provider that takes price into account. One survey of insured patients found that more than 80% wanted to discuss costs with their doctor, and 75% of patients reported they wanted their physician to consider out-of-pocket costs before making decisions for their care.[66] This kind of consultation between patient and provider reflects the

---

[65] A.D. Sinaiko et al., *Cost-Sharing Obligations, High-Deductible Health Plan Growth, and Shopping for Health Care Enrollees with Skin in the Game*. 176 JAMA INTERNAL MEDICINE 3, 395–97 (2016).

[66] N.B. Henrikson et al., *Communication with Physicians about Health Care Costs: Survey of an Insured Population*, 21 THE PERMANENTE J. 2, 16–070 (2017).

most complete form of informed consent, known as shared decision-making, in which the provider and patient jointly consider all of the relevant information about a particular treatment decision – including the costs, risks, and benefits of various treatment options – and use that information to make a treatment choice that best reflects the patient's preferences.[67] The same survey that demonstrated that patients want their doctors to consider costs found that less than half of the surveyed patients could find information about healthcare costs when needed.[68] Since primary care physicians occupy a sentinel role in connecting patients to other services, they can successfully steer patients to lower-cost facilities and providers, and offer guidance on lower-cost alternatives *if* they have access to a particular patient's insurance network, pricing, and cost-sharing obligations when recommending treatment.

Implementation of this kind of sophisticated interaction, however, faces many challenges. Foremost among them is that providers need price information that is patient, procedure, provider, and plan specific at the time of decision-making, i.e., during a patient's appointment. Few providers know what their patients will have to pay for the care they recommend. Currently, physicians often struggle to find out if a particular provider is in a patient's insurance network at the time a referral is made, so developing tools that give providers the necessary detailed information through coordinated infrastructure and interoperability between electronic medical records (EMRs) and insurers will require substantial systematic changes. However, health systems, especially those with an insurance arm, have begun offering providers such information via EMRs, and data reporting practices to APCDs could help facilitate the integration of price and insurance information into EMRs. Even if EMRs could systematically incorporate patient insurance information, provider network lists and information on which providers currently accept new patients would need to be consistently updated to reflect accurate information, so that patients do not inadvertently seek treatment from an out-of-network provider.

---

[67] Jaime S. King & Benjamin Moulton, *Rethinking Informed Consent: The Case for Shared Medical Decision- Making*, 32 AM. J. L. & MED. 429 (2006).

[68] Henrikson, *supra* note 66.

Further, the short duration of most physician visits, typically 15 minutes, limits the amount of time that can be spent on treatment choice and provider selection. Engaging a patient in a meaningful discussion about the potential risks and benefits, including financial risks and benefits, of different treatment options requires time, and providers should be paid for providing this service.

Payers

Payers for healthcare in the U.S., mostly insurers and employers, also have much to gain from increased price transparency. Approximately half of Americans receive their health insurance through their employer,[69] and as a main conduit to healthcare, employers have a strong incentive to steer their employers to high-value, lower-priced care. Employers provide health insurance to their employees by either selecting an insurance provider and contributing to premiums or by self-insuring their patients and paying directly for their care, often through a third-party administrator. When choosing an insurance plan, employers need information on the premiums, benefit design, breadth of the provider network, and the cost of services when employees must go outside of the network. When self-insuring, employers need data on the negotiated prices that health plans pay for a wide range of services to ensure they are obtaining reasonable rates. They also need information on the size of the provider network needed to ensure that patients can stay in-network for most care. Employers must have a sense of the range of rates for out-of-network care to predict their overall exposure. Having access to an APCD to analyze benchmarks for insurer negotiated rates would prove very helpful to employers seeking to self-insure their employees.

While insurers generally have access to the rates they negotiate with providers, they can also benefit from having access to benchmarks for insurer negotiated rates in a particular geographic area when negotiating their own rates. While making negotiated rates entirely transparent presents

---

[69] *Health Insurance Coverage of the Total Population*, KFF.ORG, https://www.kff.org/other/state-indicator/total-population/?currentTimeframe=0&sortModel=%7B%22colId%22:%22Location%22,%22sort%22:%22asc%22%7D (last visited July 14, 2018).

some risks of price collusion,[70] using claims data from an APCD to establish average pricing benchmarks for average to high quality providers should encourage, rather than threaten competition. Further, health plans can benefit from being able to encourage patients to select higher-value/lower-cost providers through tiering and reference pricing tools. Price transparency initiatives that prohibit anti-tiering/anti-steering contract provisions also can facilitate use of those tools.

Policymakers

Finally, policymakers probably have the most to gain from improved transparency of healthcare prices. As noted above, state governments have shown a great deal of interest in obtaining healthcare price data for a variety of uses. States can use healthcare claims data reported to an APCD to examine the drivers of healthcare costs over time, the effectiveness of various reform efforts, the impact of mergers, acquisitions, and other affiliations on healthcare price and quality, and other factors that might hinder competition and efficiency in the healthcare market. For example, Oregon recently published a report summarizing 54 use cases for its APCD, the Oregon All-Payer All-Claims Database.[71] Identifying Oregon's APCD as "an integral component of the state's ongoing healthcare improvement efforts," the report outlined numerous uses for the APCD data in analyzing and monitoring healthcare spending and cost trends, healthcare delivery system performance, healthcare utilization, population health, disease prevention, and insurance coverage.[72] Oregon, Colorado, and Maryland have used their APCD data to analyze geographic variations in price and utilization of healthcare services to detect unwarranted variations due to overutilization and market consolidation.[73]

---

[70] Erin C. Fuse Brown & Jaime S. King, *The Double-Edged Sword of Health Care Integration: Consolidation and Cost Control*, 92 IND. L. J. 55 (2016).

[71] OREGON ALL-PAYER ALL-CLAIMS DATABASE USE CASE DOCUMENT (2017), https://www.oregon.gov/oha/HPA/ANALYTICS/APAC%20Page%20Docs/APAC-Use-Cases.pdf.

[72] *Id.*

[73] A. COSTELLO ET AL., APCD COUNCIL, INFORMING HEALTH SYSTEMS CHANGE - USE OF ALL-PAYER CLAIMS DATABASES (2018), https://www.apcdcouncil.org/publication/informing-health-system-change-use-all-payer- claims-databases.

Massachusetts' APCD provides essential information to the Massachusetts Health Policy Commission to track healthcare spending trends and inform policy and legal decisions regarding consolidation and payment reform.[74] Finally, New York views its developing APCD, the NYS Connector, as a central hub of health information that will collect and synthesize all varieties of health data from the entire state. According to the New York Department of Health, "the APD [all payer database] is creating new capability within the Department, including more advanced and comprehensive analytics to support decision-making, policy development, and research, while enhancing data security by protecting patient privacy through encryption and de-identification of potentially identifying information."[75] Perhaps state health policy experts, Joel Ario and Kevin McAvey, said it best in their recent Health Affairs Blog post, "APCDs are very much a work in progress, with tremendous unrealized potential."[76]

Legal Barriers to Price Transparency

Yet a range of laws and contractual provisions currently hinder the potential of APCDs and other price transparency initiatives. Many states currently lack access to a complete set of claims data in their APCDs because federal laws, trade secret protections, and contract provisions limit what data they can demand from insurers. First and foremost, the Federal Employee Retirement Income Security Act of 1974 (ERISA) preempts any state law that "relates to an employee benefit plan."[77] ERISA's preemptive reach is limited by the "savings clause" which saves all laws that regulate insurance from preemption,[78] but ERISA does not deem self-insured

---

[74] *Massachusetts Health Policy Commission*, MASS.GOV, https://www.mass.gov/orgs/ massachusetts-health-policy- commission (last visited July 14, 2018).

[75] *New York State All Payer Database*, HEALTH.NY.GOV, https://www.health. ny.gov/technology/all_payer_database/ (last visited July 14, 2018).

[76] Ario & McAvey, *supra* note 13.

[77] ERISA § 514(a) (1974); 29 U.S.C. § 1144(a) (2006).

[78] *Kentucky Ass'n of Health Plans v. Miller*, 538 U.S. 329, 341-42 (2003). The savings clause will save state insurance regulations from preemption so long as they are "specifically

employer plans to constitute insurance for purposes of regulation. Therefore, ERISA preempts any state insurance law that relates to an employee benefit plan provided by a self-insured employer.[79] Consequently, many state transparency laws that target health plans do not apply to self-insured employers' plans, including laws requiring reporting or disclosure of healthcare claims data, drug pricing methodologies, provider network status, and billing information.

Most cripplingly, in 2015, the Supreme Court in *Gobeille v. Liberty Mutual Insurance Co.* held that ERISA preempts state APCD reporting requirements with respect to self-insured employer health benefit plans.[80] Specifically, self-insured employers and their third party administrators, which cover approximately two-thirds of all workers with employer-based health insurance, are exempt from submitting their claims data to the APCD, significantly limiting the number of plans that must report to the APCD and the percentage of employee claims data included in the database. As such, the loss of self-insured employees' claims data deprives state APCDs from having the essential information needed to provide robust analysis on healthcare cost, quality, utilization, and geographic variations within the state.

Second, as noted above, providers and insurers often include specific provisions in their contracts designed to keep healthcare prices secret, such as "gag clauses" or anti-tiering/anti-steering provisions. These types of contract provisions greatly hinder patients' ability to choose high-value services, and policymakers' ability to know and understand how to best reform the healthcare system. States have passed laws prohibiting these and other similar provisions in provider-insurer contracts, but the impact of these laws has been limited due to claims that negotiated healthcare prices constitute trade secrets.

Third, providers and insurers have successfully used trade secrets protections to prevent disclosure of negotiated healthcare price information in the absence of the contract provisions above. Historically, the states

---

directed at entities engaged in insurance," and the state law "substantially affect[s] the risk pooling arrangement between the insurer and the insured."

[79] 29 U.S.C. § 1144(b)(2)(B) (2006).

[80] *Gobeille v. Liberty Mutual Insurance Co.*, 136 S. Ct. 936 (2015).

have governed trade secret laws, but Congress passed the federal Defend Trade Secrets Act of 2016 (DTSA) to establish a floor for trade secrets protection. The DTSA allows businesses and individuals to keep information confidential if 1) "the owner has taken reasonable measures to keep such information secret"; and 2) "the information derives independent economic value, actual or potential, from not being generally known to, and not being readily ascertainable through proper means by, another person who can obtain economic value from the disclosure or use of the information."[81] Some states, like California, Illinois, and Oregon have broader protections of trade secrets that would enable more information to constitute a trade secret.

Historically, courts did not consider prices eligible for trade secret protections, but in our modern economy where business-to-business transactions are more common, this question is not so straightforward. Many healthcare organizations now claim trade secrets protections to avoid disclosure of their negotiated prices, rebates, discounts, and other pricing information. This jealous guarding of prices compromises the decision-making of nearly every stakeholder in the healthcare market and contributes significantly to the ever-rising price of healthcare goods and services. Ironically, no court has affirmatively decided that negotiated healthcare prices constitute a trade secret.[82] Trade secret cases are highly fact specific, such that even if a court found in a particular case that the confidentiality of such prices should be protected, it would not be generalizable to other cases. Yet, the mere claim that negotiated price information constitutes a trade secret has seemingly been sufficient to stop many who seek the data from continuing to do so or taking the issue to court, allowing provider and insurer organizations to use legal protections to avoid disclosure of information that has the potential to lower their revenues.

---

[81] The Defend Trade Secrets Act, 18 U.S.C.A. § 1839(3) (2016).

[82] A number of courts have discussed how negotiated price lists may be considered trade secrets, but none have ruled squarely on the issue. *See, e.g.*, *Synthes, Inc. v. Emerge Med., Inc.*, 25 F. Supp. 3d 617, 706 (E.D. Pa. 2014), *In re Maxxim Med. Grp., Inc.*, 434 B.R. 660, 669 (Bankr. M.D. Fla. 2010), *Emergency Care Research Inst. v. Guidant Corp.*, No. CIV.A. 06-1898, 2007 WL 2702455, at *5 (E.D. Pa. Sept. 12, 2007) and *Emergency Care Research Inst. v. Guidant Corp.*, No. 06-1898, 2006 WL 3541776, at *3 (E.D. Pa. Dec. 5, 2006).

Ultimately, ERISA, contract provisions, and trade secret laws form a formidable obstruction to price transparency in healthcare that require federal intervention.

What Can Congress Do?

For transparency initiatives to achieve their full effect at the state level, the federal government must make changes. Despite the need for federal policy to maximize healthcare transparency efforts, policymakers should craft changes to preserve state flexibility and innovation. Fortunately, Congress, more than any other entity, has the ability to address the most significant barriers to price transparency in healthcare and maximize the tremendous untapped potential of existing state initiatives, in particular APCDs.

1. Address ERISA Preemption Challenges

APCDs have the greatest potential of any price transparency initiative to inform consumers and policymakers in ways that can help control healthcare costs. Unfortunately, following the *Gobeille* decision to allow ERISA preemption of state APCD reporting requirements as applied to self-insured employer plans, many data reporters have reduced or ceased their submission of healthcare claims data to state APCDs, depriving state governments, researchers, and the public from access to essential information on healthcare costs, quality, and utilization.[83]

The omission of self-insured employer claims data greatly limits the accuracy and utility of APCDs. Essentially for health policy analysts, trying to analyze the healthcare landscape using an APCD without the self-insured employer population is akin to trying to use GoogleMaps with one-third of the roads missing – you don't have the whole picture. Enabling

---

[83] *See* NATIONAL ACADEMY FOR STATE HEALTH POLICY, COMMENTS ON DEPARTMENT OF LABOR NOTICE OF PROPOSED RULEMAKING 1 (2016), https://www.dol.gov/sites/default/files/ebsa/laws-and-regulations/rules-and-regulations/public-comments/1210-AB63/00030.pdf.

APCDs to collect the full set of healthcare claims data would dramatically increase the utility and reliability of these initiatives.

Congress can pursue several paths to relieving the burden of ERISA preemption on APCDs. It could pass legislation creating a federal APCD that required reporting on all claims from all healthcare payers. While a federal APCD would standardize reporting requirements, streamline, and simplify reporting mechanisms, and create one complete dataset for the entire country, such an initiative would further entrench the federal government's role in healthcare and require significant human and capital resources. A federal APCD would also fail to capitalize on the investment made by nearly half the states to develop state APCDs.

Rather than reinvent the wheel, Congress should invest its efforts in facilitating the already significant strides made by state APCDs. The most effective and direct manner of doing so would be to amend ERISA to narrow preemption to exclude state health regulations that do not unduly burden ERISA's goal of uniformity for employer-based benefit plans, while also granting states sufficient flexibility to achieve their health reform goals.[84] Amending ERISA's preemption scheme to replace broad preemption with conflict preemption would permit the states to experiment with a variety of health reform proposals, including price transparency initiatives, while permitting ERISA to preempt any state law that directly conflicts with the federal law.[85]

Alternatively, Congress could pass legislation that affirms the Department of Labor's authority to collect healthcare claims data from ERISA plans and allow them to partner with state APCDs under ERISA § 506, such that the Department of Labor could require ERISA plans to submit claims data to state APCDs.[86] For states that have not yet created an

---

[84] Erin C. Fuse Brown & Jaime S. King, *ERISA as a Barrier for State Health Care Transparency Efforts*, TRANSPARENCY IN HEALTH AND HEALTH CARE (Holly Fernandez Lynch, I. Glenn Cohen, & Barbara Evans eds., Cambridge University Press, forthcoming 2019) (manuscript at 10-11), https://ssrn.com/abstract=3214173.

[85] Elizabeth Y. McCuskey, *Body of Preemption: Health Law Traditions and the Presumption Against Preemption*, 89 TEMP. L. REV. 95, 103 (2016); Erin C. Fuse Brown & Ameet Sarpatwari, *Removing ERISA's Impediment to State Health Reform*, 378 N. Eng. J. Med. 5, 7 (2018).

[86] 29 U.S.C. § 1136 (1996).

APCD, the Department could require ERISA plans to submit claims data to a third party contracted to perform the APCD functions for those states, similar to the federal marketplace created by the Patient Protection and Affordable Care Act of 2010. The Department of Labor could facilitate the collection of this additional claims data with minimal financial investment and also develop the ability to request reports from the state APCDs on claim information from employee benefit plans.[87] On the other hand, this approach would leave ERISA's broader preemption scheme in place, which would still hinder other state transparency initiatives like surprise billing protections, pharmacy benefit transparency laws, and anti-tiering and anti-steering prohibitions, making a direct amendment of ERISA the preferred approach for promoting price transparency initiatives overall.

Under either approach, Congress should require that state APCDs request claims data in a standardized manner to minimize the burden for multi-state employers and to facilitate data comparisons across states. State APCDs have already developed and agreed upon a standardized set of healthcare claim and related data that can be collected from all health plans – the Common Data Layout.[88] The Common Data Layout creates a uniform system of reporting across all state APCDs that will ease the reporting burden on employers, third-party administrators, and insurance companies, satisfy ERISA's uniformity requirements, and facilitates analysis of claims data across states. Further, the depth of information reported in the Common Data Layout could strengthen the Department of Labor's ability to monitor ERISA plans well beyond any information the Department currently collects.

Overall, addressing ERISA preemption of state health reform laws is *the* most important action Congress could take at this time to promote price transparency to bring down healthcare costs, but additional actions by Congress could also further illuminate healthcare prices.

---

[87] *See* Fuse Brown & King, *supra* note 84, at 8-9.

[88] *See* NATIONAL ACADEMY FOR STATE HEALTH POLICY, COMMENTS ON DEPARTMENT OF LABOR NOTICE OF PROPOSED RULEMAKING (2016), https://www.dol.gov/sites/default/files/ebsa/laws-and-regulations/rules-and-regulations/public-comments/1210-AB63/00030.pdf.

2. Encourage Consumer Pricing Shopping Initiatives

Congress should seek to encourage consumer price shopping initiatives like reference pricing, rewards, and tiered networks to provide patients with further incentives to select high-value/lower-priced providers. Congress could promote reference pricing by implementing reference pricing schemes into Medicare and funding pilot projects to test reference pricing in a variety of settings. Congress could also facilitate insurers' attempts to signal lower-priced providers to patients by prohibiting anti-tiering/anti-steering provisions in contracts or prohibiting them in ERISA plan contracts.

3. Create a Public Interest Exemption to Trade Secrets

Trade secrets protections were designed to encourage and protect innovation, not protect exorbitant prices that take advantage of consumers, bankrupt businesses, and bleed government coffers. Congress should pass a public interest exemption to the Defend Trade Secrets Act of 2016 that clearly establishes that trades secret protections will not apply to information being kept secret in ways that harm the public's interest. In the case of negotiated healthcare prices, keeping negotiated rates secret from competitors in highly concentrated markets where disclosure might drive costs up might serve the public interest, but keeping those same rates secret from the government, employers who pay them, or consumers would not. Evaluation of this standard would be a highly fact-specific analysis, performed on a case by case basis, yet it would provide a clear opportunity to better define the specific contours of trade secret protections in healthcare and raise questions about whether trade secrets protections apply to all or any negotiated healthcare prices.

4. Mandate Interoperability of Electronic Medical Records Systems

Similar to the Common Data Layout, Congress should require manufacturers of electronic medical records and insurance companies to establish uniform standards of interoperability and data reporting practices, such that a patient's insurance information can load into a provider's electronic medical record to enable the provider to access meaningful network, out-of-pocket cost, and quality information for patients when making provider and medical service referrals during appointments. Placing relevant cost information into the hands of both patients and providers when they are selecting a treatment or provider will significantly increase the odds that patients will incorporate such information into their healthcare choices.

5. Develop Billing Codes to Pay for Physician Time for Shared Decision-Making

Congress should develop billing codes and other payment mechanisms within Medicare to pay for physician time in discussing treatment selection, including information on which providers are "in-network" and what the cost to the patient would be of different treatment choices. Shared decision-making that includes a discussion of the out-of-pocket costs to the patient not only encourages physicians to provide a robust form of informed consent to patients, but it also has the added benefits of encouraging patients to shop for healthcare services and potentially decreasing overutilization of services that patients would not choose if they knew all the risks and benefits.

Thank you for your time and your consideration of these important issues.

APPENDIX A: 2018 LEGISLATIVE SESSION

During the 2018 legislative session, state legislatures have attempted to pass laws related to healthcare price and quality transparency. In 2018 the legislatures have focused particularly on lowering drug prices, and as such, have constructed their legislation to target drug manufacturers, pharmacy benefits managers (PBMs), formularies, and other pharmaceutical-related entities and tools. The vast majority of these bills target consumers' access to healthcare price and quality information, rather than other stakeholders.

Focus of Bill*	Number of Bills Introduced in 2018**	Number Passed in 2018**	Number Died in 2018**
Pharmacy Gag Clauses, Clawback Prohibitions, and Mandatory Disclosure of Cheaper Drug Alternatives	55	25	17
Price Comparison (Right to Shop, the Right to Know, and Transparency Website/Tools)	46	5	23
Prohibition on Price Gouging	43	2	21
"Pricing Report" Laws (Mandatory Disclosure of Drug Prices, Increase in Costs, or Pricing Mechanisms)	41	8	16
Surprise and/or Balance Billing Laws	34	7	15
All Payer Claims Databases (APCD)	9	2	4
Reference Pricing Laws	8	2	4
Chargemaster Laws	4	0	3
Price/Claim Request	3	0	3

* Some categories of transparency bills not included in this summary as there are too few bills or do not specifically target price/quality, though they may impact either.

** All data as of July 3, 2018.

Mr. HARPER. Thank you very much, Dr. King.

And the chair will now recognize Dr. Chernew for 5 minutes for purposes of his opening statement.

STATEMENT OF MICHAEL CHERNEW

Mr. CHERNEW. Thank you very much, Chairman Harper, Ranking Member DeGette, members and staff. Thank you for the opportunity to speak with you today about price transparency in healthcare.

Before I launch into the main thrust of my comments I would like to emphasize that as an economist I believe strongly in markets. Well-functioning markets require buyers to effectively shop for the combination of price and quality that best meets their needs. And in the market for medical services, buyers, in this case patients, do not have the necessary information.

For that reason, one would think that efforts to promote price transparency in healthcare would be able to significantly lower the cost and perhaps improve the quality of care. In fact, this logic has spawned the creation of numerous transparency initiatives and tools, launched several innovative companies. All of the major insurers that I'm aware of have some price transparency tools—not all are great—as do many other vendors in several states who are pursuing transparency-related programs.

Although there are a few studies that suggest transparency initiatives may be helpful, such as the one in New Hampshire, they've only had a modest impact on the spending for some services, at best. Overall, the evidence, unfortunately, suggests that the impact of transparency has been minimal.

This reflects several institutional features of healthcare. First, healthcare is complex. Any course of treatment or diagnostic pathway is comprised of many individual services. An accurate price quote requires knowing the exact service. This is complex.

For example, there are over 50 codes for CT scans. In some cases it is even unknowable because the exact service delivered may change during the course of treatment based on clinical information that arises during that treatment. Moreover, the fees to the hospital and the physician are often separate. To get an accurate price, they have to be combined. This makes it hard, particularly for providers, to provide the information.

Imagine when shopping for a car consumers could only get the average price of a specific car, and that the actual price that they would pay depended on who put them together and the customer's employer. The information would be of limited value.

Most transparency tools seek ways around this, but so far there have not been great successes.

Second, physicians are central to almost all consequential decisions in healthcare. Physician recommendations about where to seek care appropriately carry enormous weight. As a result, few patients shop for care. In our work, we find around 10 to 15 percent of patients use transparency tools when offered. This result seems pretty standard in the literature. While it's certainly true that patients can question or even ignore their physician's referral recommendations, few do.

Third, consolidation in healthcare markets limits choice and, thus, competition in some markets. Specifically, competitive forces can only work when there are competing firms. As markets have consolidated, the potential for transparency or shopping more broadly diminishes.

Finally, insurance distorts choices. Patients fundamentally care about what they pay out of pocket. The out-of-pocket price will depend on the details of the patient's insurance plan and will change over time depending on things like whether they've met their deductible. As a result, one cannot accurately quote an out-of-pocket price without knowing details about the patient's health plan and how much they've often already spent, often for specific services. This implies that insurers are best suited to provide transparency information and, as noted, many do, although, as we've mentioned, with relatively little impact.

I do not mean to imply that transparency, or more generally price shopping for medical services, cannot work. Very simplified indicators such as flagging high-priced providers, as happened in some tiered insurance products can help, particularly when tied to benefit design. Moreover, transparency can have an impact even if it does not alter consumer behavior. The widespread availability of data may shame high-priced providers to lower their prices, particularly when journalists have access.

There's some evidence that this can be salient in healthcare. However, one has to proceed with caution, caution because it's also possible that widespread availability of information could alter the negotiation dynamics in other ways, leading to higher prices for some patients. Because payers negotiate price discounts with providers, if forced to reveal those discounts the providers may be more reticent to offer them. And there's some evidence of that in markets outside of healthcare.

So, where does this leave us? I'm generally supportive of the initiatives, particularly the private sector ones that simplify the information and focus on out-of-pocket prices. I'm more skeptical about public sector initiatives that entail new mandates on providers to provide data because it's particularly hard to get that data right. I worry it will not substantially improve the system, and may impose administrative costs.

There is certainly a lot we do not know. And while there may be deleterious unintended consequences, most evidence is either neutral or positive, and I think the shaming effect may be important in the most egregious cases. Moreover, states are experimenting in many ways, which should be allowed to play out.

So, there are a few fundamental things the Federal Government could support those efforts.

The first, as was mentioned, support the ERISA exemption or get rid of the ERISA exemption.

Providing financial support for All Payer Claims Databases could be a wise investment.

And providing more funding to AHRQ or other federal agencies to study what is actually working.

We have a lot of problems in healthcare, and I very much applaud your efforts to seek a solution. But please do not let transparency distract you from other strategies such as supporting alternative payment models or addressing adverse selection in the individual markets of healthcare that may be more impactful.

Thank you.

[The prepared statement of Mr. Chernew follows:]

Testimony of: Michael Chernew, Examining State Efforts to Improve Transparency in Health Care Costs for Consumers, Subcommittee on Oversight and Investigations, Committee on Energy and Commerce, U.S. House of Representatives, Tuesday, July 17, 2018

Main Points

- Well-functioning markets require well informed consumers.
- Consumers in health care markets are poorly informed and health care markets do not function well.
- It is logical therefore to assume that improving information in health care markets would support lower prices and better quality
- However, evidence suggests transparency initiatives that improve information in health care will not have a significant impact, though there are some clinical areas (e.g., imaging) where research is more positive. The reason for the limited broad impact is that other aspects of health care markets limit their effectiveness
  - Health care services are purchased in very fragmented units
  - Patients defer to physicians
  - Some markets have too few providers to be considered competitive
  - Insurance masks true price differentials
- Nevertheless, policy makers can take some action to support greater competition, these include
  - Requiring ERISA plans to submit data to All Payer Claims Databases
  - Providing financial support to APCDs
- Funding greater research on competition and competitive strategies

Testimony

Chairman Harper, ranking minority member Degette, members and staff, thank you very much for the opportunity to speak with you today about price transparency in health care. I am going to confine my remarks to transparency in the context of medical services, excluding prescription drugs or insurance. This is only because the market for insurance is completely different than that for health care services and the prescription drug market has unique issues and complexities.

Before I launch into the main thrust of my comments, I would like to emphasize that as an economist I believe strongly in the merits of markets. Moreover, I suspect that you have asked me here today because you, correctly, recognize that markets for medical services are not working well. This is part because well-functioning markets require buyers to effectively shop for the combination of price and quality that best meets their needs and in the market for medical services buyers—in this case patients—do not have the necessary information.

Taken together, the logic outlined above would suggest that efforts to promote price transparency in health care would be able to significantly lower the cost, and perhaps improve the quality, of care. In fact, this logic has spawned the creation of numerous transparency initiatives and launched several innovative companies. All of the major insurers I am aware of have transparency tools, as do many other vendors and several states are pursuing transparency related programs.

Although there are a few studies that suggest transparency initiatives, such as New Hampshire, can have a modest impact on spending for some services,[89] overall, the evidence, unfortunately, has not been kind to these initiatives. Many studies, including several of my own and those of my

---

[89] http://www.economics.illinois.edu/seminars/documents/Brown.Pdf; Whaley C, Schneider Chafen J, Pinkard S, et al. Association between availability of health service prices and payments for these services. *JAMA*. 2014;312(16):1670-1676. doi: 10.1001/jama.2014.13373.

colleagues, find that transparency has minimal, if any impact on the market.[90] This reflects several institutional features of health care.

First, health care is complex. Any course of treatment (or diagnostic pathway) is comprised of many individual services. For example, there are 10 codes for office visits and 56 for CT scans (based on the CPT code list CMS released in Nov 2017).[91] If one wants to know the price of a service, one would need to specify the exact service and that is hard. In some cases, it is even unknowable because the exact service delivered may change during the course of a test or procedure based on clinical information that arises. Though this complexity can be minimized by reporting averages for broader service groups, many providers are often involved in care delivery and each has a different price. For example, a surgery will include different fees to the hospital and surgeon. The hospital will likely not know the surgeon's fee and the surgeon will not know the hospital fees.

I am aware of several website that support shopping for other important items such as cars. But imagine those websites could only provide data on specific parts and the customer had to know which were needed and how well they would work together. That would diminish, if not destroy the usefulness of such shopping tools. In addition to the complexity arising from the fragmented way in which we buy care, any given provider is paid a different amount from different insurers. In one study we found that large insurers paid 21% less than smaller ones.[92] Therefore, to quote an accurate price, one must know the patient's insurer (and maybe even their exact health plan). All of this complexity makes seemingly simple goals, like requiring providers to post or provide accurate price quotes, difficult.

Second, the physicians are central to almost all consequential decisions in health care. Patients trust their physicians to guide them through the episode of care, laying out alternatives and recommending treatments. Physician recommendations about where to seek care carry enormous

---

[90] Desai S, Hatfield LA, Hicks AL, Chernew ME, Mehrotra A. Association Between Availability of a Price Transparency Tool and Outpatient Spending. *JAMA*. 2016;315(17):1874-1881.

[91] https://www.cms.gov/Medicare/Fraud-and-Abuse/PhysicianSelfReferral/List_of_Codes.html.

[92] Roberts ET, Chernew ME, McWilliams JM. Market Share Matters: Evidence of Insurer and Provider Bargaining Over Prices. HEALTH AFFAIRS 36, NO. 1 (2017): 141–148.

weight. As a result, few patients shop for care. In our work we find that around 10% to 15% percent of patients used a transparency tool when offered.[93] This result seems pretty standard in the literature.[94] While it is certainly true that patients can question, or even ignore, their physician's referral recommendations, few do.

Third, consolidation in health care markets limits choice, and thus competition, in some markets. Specifically, competitive forces can only work when there are competing firms. Gaynor and colleagues (2015) report that between 1990 and 2006, the proportion of metropolitan statistical areas (MSAs) with "highly concentrated" hospital markets increased from 65 percent to 80 percent.[95] Likewise, Capps and colleagues (2017) report that 22 percent of physician markets in 2013 were highly concentrated.[96] Moreover, hospitals are increasingly buying physician practices further diminishing competition.[97]

Finally, insurance distorts choices. Some patients may care about the total price of care, but most fundamentally care about what they pay out of pocket. Often insurance masks the true cost of care because patients pay just a fraction, if any, of the price. Very sick patients, who spend the most, are the most likely to be largely protected once they hit their out of pocket maximum. Even if they do have to pay, the price will depend on the details of patients' insurance plan and will change over time depending on things like if they have met their deductible. As a result, one cannot quote an

---

93 Desai S, Hatfield LA, Hicks AL, Sinaiko AD, Chernew ME, Cowling D, Gautam S, Wu SJ Mehrotra A. Offering A Price Transparency Tool Did Not Reduce Overall Spending Among California Public Employees And Retirees. Health Aff (Millwood). 2017 Aug 1;36(8):1401-1407.

94 Desai S, Hatfield LA, Hicks AL, Chernew ME, Mehrotra A. Association Between Availability of a Price Transparency Tool and Outpatient Spending. *JAMA*. 2016;315(17):1874-1881. Mehrotra A, Dean KM, Sinaiko AD, Sood N. Americans Support Price Shopping For Health Care, But Few Actually Seek Out Price Information. Health Aff (Millwood). 2017 Aug 1;36(8):1392-1400.

95 Gaynor, M., K. Ho, and R. J. Town. 2015. The industrial organization of health-care markets. *Journal of Economic Literature* 53(2):235–284.

96 Capps, CoryC., David D. Dranove, and Christopher C. Ody. 2017. "Physician practice consolidation driven by small acquisitions, so antitrust agencies have few tools to intervene." Health Affairs 36(9):1556-–1563.

97 Neprash, Hannah H. T., Michael M. E. Chernew, Andrew A. L. Hicks, Teresa T. Gibson, and J. Michael M. McWilliams. 2015. "Association of financial integration between physicians and hospitals with commercial health care prices." JAMA Internal Medicine 175(12):1932-–1939.

accurate out of pocket price without knowing details of a patients plan AND how much they have already spent on care (and often on which types of services). This implies that insurers are best suited to provide transparency information, and, as noted, many do, though most evidence suggests with little impact even in markets where shopping is possible.

I do not mean to imply that transparency, and more generally price shopping for medical services, cannot work. However, even in areas where we might assume it would work well, such as Lasik surgery, evidence is less promising.[98] Perhaps shopping will work better in areas where there is greater patient responsibility for the price, less reliance on referrals, services that are less complex and, such as in the case of durable medical equipment, involve repeated purchases. Some of the most positive evidence focuses on imaging. Yet, I consider these areas exceptions rather than the rule.

I should also note that transparency may have an impact even if it does not alter consumer behavior. The widespread availability of data may shame high price providers to lower their prices (particularly when journalists have access). There is some evidence that this effect can be salient in healthcare.[99]

However, one must proceed with caution because it is also possible that widespread availability of information could alter negotiation dynamics in other ways leading to higher prices for some, likely many, patients.[100] This is because payers negotiate discounts with providers. If forced to reveal those discounts health care providers be more reticent to offer them. In fact, there is some evidence, from outside of health care, to support the perverse impact of posting prices.[101]

So where does all of this leave us? Believe it or not, I am generally supportive of transparency initiatives. They are important as we move to newer, innovative benefit designs that attempt to help patients shop. They

---

98 http://www.hschange.org/CONTENT/862/?topic=topic01#note8.

99 https://www.chcf.org/wp-content/uploads/2017/12/PDF-MovingMarketsNewHampshire.pdf.

100 Cutler D, Dafny L. Designing Transparency Systems for Medical Care Prices. N Engl J Med 2011; 364:894-895.

101 Albaek, Svend, Peter Mollgaard, and Per B Overgaard, "Government-Assisted Oligopoly Coordination? A Concrete Case," *Journal of Industrial Economics*, Vol. 45 (1997): 429-43.

need not be tremendously detailed and may provide broad categories of price (and/ or quality, which I admitted have not emphasized enough). For example, they can label providers high value or preferred. Simpler information is easier for patients to digest and act upon.

As I mentioned at the onset, I believe in markets and the commercial insurance market is responding by providing transparency tools (and redesigning plans and networks) to encourage shopping.

I am more skeptical about public sector initiatives that entail new mandates on providers to provide data because it is particularly hard to provide the right data. I worry that it will not substantially improve the system and may impose administrative costs. I worry that some transparency advocates, in their zeal to help markets work, will override what markets are doing. That said, there is certainly a lot we do not know. While there may be deleterious unintended consequences, there is some positive evidence and I think the shaming effect may be important in the most egregious cases. Moreover, states are experimenting in many ways and there are ways the federal government could support that. For example, requiring ERISA covered health plans to submit data to all payer claims databases (APCDs), which the supreme court, in *Gobeille v. Liberty Mutual Insurance Company*, ruled the states could not do. Providing financial support to APCDs could be a wise investment. Finally, it is clear that healthcare is sufficiently complex that our intuition about how consumers and markets will behave may not be correct. Mine was not. Supporting evidence generation with research funds through AHRQ or other federal mechanisms could help us steer the most productive path forward.

We have a lot of problems in healthcare, I very much applaud your efforts to seek solutions. But please do not let transparency distract you from other strategies, such as supporting alternative payment models, or addressing adverse selection in the individual market for health care, that may be more impactful.

Sincerely,
Michael E. Chernew, Ph.D.

Mr. HARPER. Thank you both for your testimony. It is now the opportunity, the moment that you have waited for, our members get to ask questions of each of you. That will help us very much in that process. And I will now recognize myself for 5 minutes for the purpose of that. And I will start with you, if I may, Dr. King.

Obviously, it is clear that a lot of Americans struggle greatly with how to pay for their healthcare costs. And part of that is they never know how much it is going to cost until they see a bill sometime later. And as you noted in your testimony, a lot of transparency initiatives have focused on changing consumer behavior to encourage them to select lower price providers and services.

But can you elaborate on why these initiatives seem to have limited usage and have mixed results?

Ms. KING. Yes. So, I think there are largely four reasons why consumers don't tend to use these as much as we would like them to. And the first is that insurance often, the structure of insurance often insulates consumers from feeling the price, different prices for different providers.

If you pay a $20 copay every time you go to the doctor, it doesn't really matter to you what type of doctor you go to; right? So there is some function of that.

The second is that the provider relationship is really important to patients. And it turns out where we have seen price transparency work is exactly on the thing that you noted before, Chairman Harper, is on shoppable goods. We have seen some movement there, where things that people find interchangeable. Right?

So, you might go, you don't care where you go to an MRI, to have your MRI tested or have your CT scan done. Those seem likely to go to this lab or that lab, unless this lab or that lab automatically supplies the results into your electronic medical record and it goes directly to your provider. That might make a difference to you.

But, generally, those are places where people are more willing to shop.

Where they're less willing to shop is on provider, right? They want a recommendation. Let's say that you, your child, or your spouse, or your loved one just got diagnosed with cancer. Are you really going to look at a list of providers and their charges to decide where you're going to go? You're not. You're going to go to a trusted primary care physician, or a family member that's had experience with cancer and ask them who they went to and who they had a good experience for.

So, I think the reality is is that healthcare is so important that patients really want to get advice from someone they trust and not the provider. And that's really why price transparency initiatives that put pricing information that is relevant to the patient in terms of their out-of-pocket costs in the hands of the provider so it's there when they're making that decision, I think have the most, the greatest possibility of a shifting choice on the provider side.

Mr. HARPER. OK.

Ms. KING. And the last thing is that there's very, as Dr. Chernew pointed out, there's very little standardization in healthcare pricing; right? So, if you look at one, if you look at one sheet and it says, well, you can get an MRI for $300, but then you don't know if the MRI needs specific dyes or other things accompanying it, it's very hard for a patient to navigate that and to figure out what the overarching price will be for that.

Mr. HARPER. All right. Thank you very much.

Dr. Chernew, in your testimony you noted that there are several institutional features of healthcare that make it difficult for transparency alone to have a significant impact on the market. You do highlight however, that the transparency initiatives are important as we move to a newer innovative benefit designs that attempt to help patients shop.

Can you please elaborate on that point?

Mr. CHERNEW. Of course. So, let me say for those of you that don't know or may not care, I chair the Benefits Committee at Harvard University, which means I advise the provost on what we, as an employer, should do for the benefits for our workers. And we've been very worried about the variation of prices within Massachusetts, which was pointed out. And so that was painful, thank you.

So, when we think about what to do we start with how we might change our benefit designs to incent our workers to make more informed choices about providers. One cannot do that without having the relevant information available. So, if you want to do tiered network, if you want to do reference pricing, if you want to do any type of benefit design that involves incenting patients beyond a flat, say, $20 copay, it's important that you have the tools to provide information to them. In that way I think transparency is important. And you should know all of our vendors will provide such transparency tools should you decide to do that.

Mr. HARPER. Are the right to shop laws that also provide the financial incentives for consumers to choose the lower cost options perhaps, are they likely to have an impact do you think, a bigger impact on spending?

Mr. CHERNEW. I'm not familiar enough with all of all the laws, so I would defer to Dr. King. But I think that the general sense that allowing patients to shop and supporting their ability to shop when they want to I think is valuable. But because of all of the institutional features I think that alone is not really what's going to be helpful.

What we really care a lot about is even if you're not shopping you just may want to know up front what you're going to have to pay. And just getting that, which seems incredibly reasonable, is hard to do. And we're working through that.

Mr. HARPER. Thank you very much.

The chair will now recognize the ranking member of the subcommittee, Ms. DeGette, for 5 minutes.

Ms. DEGETTE. Thank you. Mr. Chairman, just to show how bipartisan this subcommittee can be, you just asked my question. So I am going to follow up on what you were talking about. And I will start with you, Dr. King.

And what I want to ask you is what percentage of healthcare costs are these things that would be negotiable to most patients, the MRI, the lab tests, issues like that? And what percentage is the things they are less likely to want to negotiate on, like physician services?

Ms. KING. I think it's a great question. And I am not, I am not a health economist. I'm not studying, somebody who studies all of that percentage, so I don't know exactly.

I know that in studies, there was a study done that looked at Anthem, and United, and some other big health insurers, and it suggested that if they used reference pricing for their shoppable items, for their laboratory tests, that they would be able to bring down costs. I think it was on the order of around 10 to 15 percent.

So I don't know the exact number of laboratories. So maybe Dr. Chernew knows that.

Ms. DEGETTE. Well, he is a health economist. Ms. KING. Yes. He may know.

Ms. DEGETTE. So I think I will ask him that.

Mr. CHERNEW. In great humility, there's a lot of things I don't know.

Ms. DEGETTE. Even though you are at Harvard?

Mr. CHERNEW. Especially because I'm at Harvard.

Ms. DEGETTE. Good answer.

So, so you don't have any idea what the percentage would be reduced?

Mr. CHERNEW. Advocates of shopping will give you a very big number, 60, 70 percent.

Ms. DEGETTE. Yes.

Mr. CHERNEW. In for realistic numbers about what really could be shopped, I think you're probably talking closer to 10 to 15 percent of services.

Ms. DEGETTE. That is the same thing Dr. King just said.

Now, now if you, if you did have increased transparency and if you could encourage patients to actually look at the sources, with physician costs even though, even though people, I mean I am not going to pick the cut-rate physician over the more expensive one that might have gotten a good reference, or whatever. But would there be some incentive for physicians to, on their own, maybe tamp down some of their rates?

Mr. CHERNEW. So, the answer is if the markets were working well there would be an incentive for physicians to change and facilities to change their prices. And you've seen some of that. I really don't associate that with transparency, I associate that with benefit design, things like reference pricing.

I also think there's evidence, we've done a lot of work on alternative payment models, which I know is not the specific subject of this hearing, but when physicians are in payment models that give them an incentive to shop——

Ms. DEGETTE. Right.

Mr. CHERNEW [continuing]. They are much more active in shopping because they will change their referral patterns if they get to keep some of the savings if they're more efficient in their referral patterns.

So, really I think transparency should be thought of as a tool that supports other impactful things as opposed to an end in and of itself.

Ms. DEGETTE. Dr. King, did you want to add to that?

Ms. KING. Yes. So, on the reference pricing point, so the way that reference pricing works is that an insurer will pick a fee that it decides that it's an amount that it's willing to pay for a particular service. And then any provider that charges above that, the patient has to pay that out of pocket.

And what the studies have shown with respect to that is that a number—there's been a decent amount of savings from patients saying they don't actually want to go to a higher-priced provider, but there's been a 30 percent reduction in provider costs overall, that they have dropped their prices to be under the reference price to get a broader volume of patients. And so that might be, that might prove to be helpful.

Ms. DEGETTE. Dr. Chernew, do you want to?

Mr. CHERNEW. I think Dr. King's referring to a study by Jamie Robinson and colleagues about a program that CalPERS did in California Anthem. There's a lot of things they did besides just reference pricing. So it's a very complicated thing. And they were a very big purchaser, which is helpful.

I think we looked at reference pricing for our employees. And one of the problems we had was if you pick a price and then the patient's responsible for the amount above that price, you actually have a lot higher bills that they have to pay.

Ms. DEGETTE. Right.

Mr. CHERNEW. Substantially higher bills. And the whole reason you're here is because you're upset, I'm upset that the patients are facing very substantial bills.

So, we are trying to find ways in our benefit design to support shopping without going through the full risk that reference pricing might impose on patients should they not shop. So, it's a complicated tradeoff.

Ms. DEGETTE. So, what did you do?

Mr. CHERNEW. We decided not to recommend reference pricing.

Ms. DEGETTE. OK.

Mr. CHERNEW. And you should know, going in I really wanted to recommend it because as an economist I thought it would be a victory.

Ms. DEGETTE. Yes. And so what it is sounding like to me is that while we can, we can work on some of these transparency issues—Dr. King, you mentioned your five items and, don't worry, they are in your testimony, too, so even though you were kind of cut short—but, but we should also look at other ways of structuring these insurance plans which may make incentives for providers versus just the patients.

Thank you. Thank you, I yield back.

Mr. HARPER. The gentlewoman yields back.

The chair will now recognize the vice chairman of this subcommittee, the gentleman from Virginia, Mr. Griffith, for 5 minutes.

Mr. GRIFFITH. Thank you very much. Appreciate you all being here today. And obviously this is a very complicated subject, and I do appreciate it.

I wish there was some way people could go in and say I have got to have this procedure and, like a car, you could say if you are getting this, the fancy wheels, then you pay more, et cetera. But it seems that that is outside of our realm right now. Although one would hope that with all these young computer whizzes coming on that somebody might be able to figure out how to plug all that in.

And I do agree that there are some things, I am going to pay more for the doctor that I know. Happy to do that, and able to do that, fortunately. Some people aren't. And so we have to try to look at some of the things that you all already talked about in relationship to insurance and getting the ability to say how much is this going to cost me out of pocket before you go forward I think is important. And you all touched on that as well.

So, you all are dealing with this huge, complicated matter. And my questions are much simpler. I have just been really concerned. We had a hearing in the Health Subcommittee where we had all the providers lined up. And it was shocking, I had heard rumors but they actually confirmed that because of the way the system currently works there are cases where you could go to your pharmacist with your insurance company and your PBM and say, I want to get this drug, how much will it cost me if I don't use my insurance? And sometimes it is less if you don't use your insurance than it is if you do use your insurance because of the complicated formulas, and so forth.

And Delegate Todd Pillion in my district out of Abingdon, Virginia, got a bill through the Virginia legislation—I heard there were 22 others this morning—that said you can't have those gag orders anymore.

Dr. King, do the states eliminating those gag orders, do we find that that make a whole lot of difference when they go to the pharmacy? Do they sometimes figure out that they are better off nothing using their insurance because of the PBMs, et cetera?

Ms. KING. Thank you. It's a great question.

So, I think a lot of these laws are new and so we haven't been able to really do the studies on them. But I think in terms of allowing pharmacists to actually say to the client at the desk, by the way, if you go outside your insurance or you get this generic you can save a lot of money, I can't, because pharmaceutical drugs in a large respect are those kinds of interchangeable drugs, interchangeable products, and so I think that that should have some substantial effect. And the idea that they were prevented from doing so by contract before is unconscionable to me. So, I think it's great.

Mr. GRIFFITH. Mr. Carter has a bill I am glad to be a cosponsor of to make that a Federal policy. And it is really interesting. I was discussing it back home and lady said, yes, that happened to my sister by accident. Her insurance company initially stated that they wouldn't pay. And so she paid for the prescription herself. Then when it came time to renew they said, oh, we changed our minds, we will pay for that particular prescription, and she found out it was more.

She called her pharmacy and said, what is this, it cost me more when I am using my insurance?

Ms. KING. Yes.

Mr. GRIFFITH. He says, yes, I can't tell you about that but if you will ask me to do it outside of your insurance you will only have to 17 instead of paying 50.

Ms. KING. Right.

Mr. GRIFFITH. And so, I think it is something we need to pass. And there are a fair number of patrons on that.

But it was clear to me that we need to look at the PBMs along with all the other things that you all are mentioning as part of the transparency. I know they serve good purpose.

But, again, Virginia on this, and it is my home State, that is why I keep referencing, but we had Delegate Keith Hodges out of Gloucester directed the State Bureau of Insurance to report to the General Assembly about how PBMs charge for their services and whether they save money or make healthcare costlier. Among the findings of the first PBM transparency report as a result of his work, mandated by that language, last year there were 152,250 payments, with total PBM markups of 3.5 million between July 1 and September 21.

The differential or spread on each claim ranged from 1 penny to $4,932.

Do you think that having more transparency and more oversight over PBMs and what they are doing—I know they work hard in some cases and save money, but in other cases they are actually costing the consumer—do you think that would help?

Ms. KING. Yes, I do.

Mr. GRIFFITH. Dr. King, you do.

Dr. Chernew, do you have an opinion?

Mr. CHERNEW. You can call me Michael, please.

Mr. GRIFFITH. Michael.

Mr. CHERNEW. I think as a matter of principle people should be able to get the information that they need. So, just on the pure principle of it.

In terms of the market demand, that gets much more complicated. I, I didn't talk about prescription drugs because a lot of the situation that you're discussing arises because of the complicated rebate rules that are going on in the prescription drug market. And those rebates both in some ways they help markets work, but in other ways, and I think more dominantly, they make it much more complicated and much more difficult to have markets work well in healthcare.

And so, I think that while we could debate conceptually what the ability, you should have the ability to negotiate, I think the fact though we live in an environment where it's just so complex for people to get the price and get simple information, they're told that by contract they're not allowed to tell them, I think it's just a matter of principle that the situation shouldn't arise, even though it may well result in some people paying more because the discount that currently the PBMs can get might be less because they don't want everybody to know when they're getting the discount. That's basically what the problem is.

Mr. GRIFFITH. All right, I appreciate it. And I think that for a lot of our folks back home, they don't understand all the big stuff. But they understand when they go to their pharmacist and they feel like they are being overcharged.

I appreciate it, and yield back.

Mr. HARPER. The gentleman yields back.

The chair will now recognize the gentlewoman from Florida, Ms. Castor, for 5 minutes.

Ms. CASTOR. Thank you, Mr. Chairman.

I want to return to what providers and insurers can do to help lower the costs through their transparency efforts. Because I think you correctly stated how folks feel, that if their doctor recommends something, I mean, it is pretty rare that a patient, a neighbor is going to go shop and do something else.

So, Dr. Chernew, you, you said, OK, alternative payment models can be one way. What else on physicians, because they play such a central role on consumer behavior?

Mr. CHERNEW. So, first let me say I really wish I could come here with some silver bullet and solve the problem. And I can't. Because anything I'm about to say is going to have potential deleterious consequences.

Most of the insurers I know, all of the insurers I actually know, are struggling to find ways to address the healthcare cost problem. It is not that insurers want healthcare spending to be high or they're not working on it.

Essentially what matters is the interaction between the patient and the physician, the treatment that's given, and the price that we pay for that. The way to address that is some combination of payment reform and benefit design. And you're seeing a ton of private sector initiatives to do that. And where we are right now is employers in the market sorting through which ones work for them in which particular ways, and we're trying to learn what works better than not.

So, alternative payment models honestly is my favorite. I'm a big believer in benefit design changes. So the evidence on high deductible health plans that are HSA coupled isn't as strong as I would like as an economist in general. There are some things that I would recommend, like the way chronic care medications are treated in the HSAs is something I think are probably a good thing to help people being able to shop. Things like that.

But there is not a specific Federal thing that one can do. And the challenge that you will face—and again I say this in a totally non-partisan way—is where the regulations should step in and stop at least the most egregious cases. Because there are some really out-of-network billing things, there are some really egregious cases that are just unconscionable that should probably be stopped by regulation. And I honestly think that transparency is not the mechanism to get at those types of things.

To the extent that the private sector can build transparency tools, which I am supportive of, and the States can try different ways through their All Payer Claims Databases, I think that is wonderful. But I think fundamentally my advice would be focus on rules to prevent the most egregious situations where people in an emergency room are paying some huge out-of-pocket thing.

Ms. CASTOR. Right.

Mr. CHERNEW. And telling them that matters. But, honestly, I would say just prevent that.

Ms. CASTOR. So and, Dr. King, your number one recommendation was on ERISA. And ERISA was a law passed in the 1970s that said, across the country you have to have certain standards.

Ms. KING. Yes.

Ms. CASTOR. So, why would that be so important for us to get into to help lower healthcare costs? You want to empower the states to do additional things I guess?

Ms. KING. So, basically ERISA, the way that it is written because it's trying to promote uniformity and place benefit plan regulation across all 50 states has a very broad preemption scheme. Which means that it will come in and negate any state law that relates to an employee benefit plan, including all the employer health plans.

Now, there is a savings clause as a part of ERISA which says that any state insurance law that directly regulates insurance will be saved from ERISA preemption. But there's the next part of ERISA says that it doesn't deem self-insured employer plans to be insurance, even though that's the way that the vast majority, or at least half of our employees get their insurance is through self-insured employer plans. Right?

So, any law that's passed by a state to regulate health insurance or employer-based insurance is going to be preempted by ERISA as it applies to about half of our employees. And ——

Ms. CASTOR. Who would oppose it?

Ms. KING. I think industry would oppose it. Right? They, they like not having regulations apply to them in that way. But it is crippling state All Payer Claims Databases, which have demonstrated that they can do a lot.

They're doing a lot with the information they have. But if they had all the claims, healthcare claims in a particular state, they could really get a handle on what's driving cost, where is competition not working, what thing, what mergers and acquisitions should or shouldn't go through.

And it also provides the foundation for every, like, for the majority of other, the other solutions we're talking about, so, allowing individuals to have better price information for what it would cost them, for putting that information into the hands of providers, I mean providers and insurers. Like, it would just sort of seed a lot of other efforts. Reference pricing would be based on that, and other things.

So, I think addressing the ERISA problem—and I have a number of ways, a number of ideas of how you could do that—I think is foundational to any sort of transparency initiative that you would propose.

Ms. CASTOR. Thank you very much. I yield back.

Mr. HARPER. The gentlewoman yields back.

The chair will now recognize the gentleman from Texas, Mr. Barton, for 5 minutes.

Mr. BARTON. Thank you, Mr. Chairman. And it is always good to have hearings like this to try to, through bipartisan basis, get facts on the table.

My first question is just kind of a general question. I have been on this committee 32 years. I have been involved with some of the major healthcare issues over a number of times. One of the most vexing issues we face is pricing drugs. And to my mind, except for the long-time over-the-counter drugs like aspirin and things of this sort, there is no rational explanation for how we price drugs.

I think the over-the-counter drugs that have been on the market for decades, in some cases hundreds of years, they are pretty much priced like any other commodity and it is cost-based, distribution-based, advertising. You pay more for Bayer aspirin than you do for the Walmart generic brand, but they are basically aspirin.

But I would like you, Dr. Chernew, to go back to the Harvard Business School and have them come up with a flow chart and explanation of how we price Lipitor, or how we price Plavix, or how we price the new stem cell-based drugs. Do either one of you want to defend the current pricing system for these, these new drugs that are coming on the market, or even try to explain it?

Mr. CHERNEW. When you said comment, I thought you were going to say comment, I was going to jump in. When you said defend I had to back off.

But I will do my best. The——

Mr. BARTON. Do it in about 30 seconds because I have got two or three questions. Give me the executive summary.

Mr. CHERNEW. New drugs provide great value. I think that is indisputable.

Mr. BARTON. I agree with that.

Mr. CHERNEW. We have a patent system that supports them.

And the drug companies charge what the market will bear. And that, fundamentally, both gets us really good drugs and creates huge amounts of problems.

And that was my 30 seconds. I'm happy to talk more.

Mr. BARTON. Well, that is pretty rational. The drug manufacturers charge what they think the market will bear. But you go through these convoluted, average wholesale pricing and 340B discount drug program.

Mr. CHERNEW. That's all just a distraction. They're basically charging what the market would bear. And because of a bunch of rules, it's much more complicated than that. And the question is how we want to support innovation and pharmaceuticals, which we want to support because it——

Mr. BARTON. We do.

Mr. CHERNEW. And that's where the problem comes in.

Mr. BARTON. Dr. King. Then I have got two more questions.

Ms. KING. I just want to interject that I think Dr. Chernew is totally right that we get, we tend to get good value for new drugs, for most of them. Where we're really not getting good value is where we've already had a drug that has been on patent, expired its patent life, and then they change a tiny little bit of this drug, get an entirely new patent, run prices up for 20 more years.

There's a lot of things that we are not getting good value for that remain in patent.

And if you want to look strongly at how to fix drug pricing, I would look at how drugs are patented and what we allow a whole re-upping on the patent.

Mr. BARTON. I think that is valid.

All right, I want to go to the very bottom line here. I have a constituent in Texas, a real estate agent who is on Medicare. And her doctor gave her a coupon for a prescription drug covered by Medicare. She took it to her pharmacist and the pharmacist said, "Great, but I can't, I can't take this coupon because you are on Medicare." Medicare doesn't take coupons.

So I got with the Congressional Research Service and some other groups and found out that for some reason when we established Medicare we don't allow senior citizens—and we started covering prescription drugs—we don't allow senior citizens to use coupons if they are under Medicare.

So, Congressman Doyle and I have got a bill, we are going to introduce it either this week or next week, that says if you are on Medicare and you have got a coupon from your doctor, you can't use them for generic drugs, but for any other drug you can. Good idea, bad idea?

Mr. CHERNEW. So, I appreciate your constituent's problems. I think the challenge is most of the time in the patent system what the market will bear is not distorted by insurance. In healthcare it's distorted by insurance. So the problem is if you take any consumer incentive away by the coupon, the actual price for the drug the market will bear goes up. And that's what the tension is, is that if you want the consumers to——

Mr. BARTON. Well, then the manufacturer doesn't have to give the coupon. If they don't give the coupon to the doctor, the doctor doesn't give it to the patient.

Mr. CHERNEW. No, the manufacturer likes giving coupons because then they charge a higher price and the insurer can't use the cost function.

Mr. BARTON. Then we should just stiff the Medicare recipients?

Mr. CHERNEW. Is my time up? I hope so.

[Laughter.]

Mr. BARTON. It is not complicated if you are an elected member of Congress and all of a sudden Medicare recipients start showing up at their town, town hall.

Mr. CHERNEW. Yes. I, I totally agree. The challenge at the core is you want the market to discipline the providers, which requires people having to pay. And when people have to pay, it turns out they don't like having to pay. And therein lies the problem with coupons and a bunch of other distortionary things.

So, I agree with you. And we'll have to have a longer conversation on how to deal with it.

Mr. BARTON. I think that is yes, he agrees with me.

Mr. HARPER. The gentleman yields back.

The chair will now recognize the gentlewoman from New York, Ms. Clarke, for 5 minutes.

Ms. CLARKE. I thank you, Chairman Harper, Ranking Member DeGette, for convening this important hearing examining state efforts to improve transparency of healthcare costs for consumers. Additionally, I want to thank our witnesses for providing your expert testimony here this morning.

This is a critical issue that is most deserving of Congress' attention as we work with industry to ensure consumers have a positive experience on their healthcare journey. In my home State of New York, since 2015 we have an out-of-network law that protects patents from surprise billing when services are performed by non-participating providers. This same law also protects New Yorkers from bills for emergency services.

The focus on transparency and consumer protection are needed so that consumers will not have to continue paying more than their usual in-network cost sharing and/or copayment amounts.

So, I have a couple of questions. Dr. King, how effective have state efforts been to ban surprise out-of-network hospital bills? And what more should we be doing to prevent this?

Ms. KING. Thank you. It's a great question.

I think surprise billing is a really important issue for just consumer protection in general. So I think that we have seen a number of different types of laws to protect consumers from surprise billing. So there are those that, as Dr. Chernew said, ban the practice outright, just say you will not be exposed, especially in emergency services, you will not be exposed to prices that are higher than your in-network copay for emergency services and other things.

And I think those are very effective. At least they're protecting the consumer. And then we allow the bigger fish in the game, the insurance companies and the providers, to hash it out over what are reasonable reimbursement rates. And that's what we have in California.

But there are others, there are lots of states that are passing laws right now that just say that a person should be informed that they may be being seen by an out-of-network provider, or that they, when they arrive at the emergency room, someone who takes care of them might be an out-of-network provider and they might experience other charges.

And I think that these laws, while well-intentioned, don't reflect accurately the reality of the patient experience. If you show up at the emergency room, you are in an emergency situation. You are signing whatever it is that you're signing and then you're going to get help. And I think that someone telling you that you may be subject to out-of-network law, out-of-network bills at that point is not that helpful for you.

So, I think we need to focus on the laws that seven states have passed that really just make it very clear that patients in these specific situations will not be subject to copays that are higher than what their in-network charges would be, and then let everybody else hash it out.

Ms. CLARKE. OK. And, Dr. Chernew, in your written testimony you note that efforts in New Hampshire have had a modest impact on healthcare spending. What was it about the reforms in New Hampshire that have enabled costs to go down, albeit slightly?

Mr. CHERNEW. So, the study by Zach Brown in Columbia is what I, who is at Columbia is what I was referring to. And they found by looking at MRIs what I consider to be a modest impact on a service where you often see impacts, like MRIs.

So I think there were some things about that. They had insurer-specific prices. They knew whether you were in your deductible or were not in your deductible, things like that.

So, I think as those laws go that's a reasonable law. I think it's a mistake to believe that doing things like that are going to solve the basic problems. And as far as I know, New Hampshire has not really solved all of the problems. Maybe there's someone here from New Hampshire.

But I think in the end of the day through their All Payer Claims Database they were able to do some things that were valuable. And to the extent that you can support the All Payer Claims Databases, I think you might be able to help on the margins the system get a bit better.

I still think private sector initiatives could have the potential to be more impactful.

Ms. CLARKE. So, Dr. King, could you describe any other promising state efforts to improve transparency of healthcare costs for their citizens?

Ms. KING. Yes. I'll comment just really briefly on New Hampshire and then I'll talk a little bit about Massachusetts as well.

So, one of the things that New Hampshire did through their All Payer Claims Database is they have a website called New Hampshire Health Costs which you can go into. And I checked it out this morning because I had heard good things about it. And basically as a, as a patient you can go there and check off this is the health insurance plan that I am in, I am in Anthem and I want to get this kind of procedure, and I want to do it with this particular provider. And they'll tell you, they'll run down the cost. And they'll run down the cost for that provider and they'll show you how it, how it compares to other providers.

Now, that doesn't tell you your specific out-of-pocket costs and it doesn't tell you where you are in your personal deductible, but I think that is more helpful than what we've seen in a lot of other states' price transparency initiatives.

Now the other state that I want to highlight here is Massachusetts. And Massachusetts has gone a long way with their All Payer Claims Databases. But they also have their Health Policy Commission, which is an arm that is designed to analyze that information and really mine the All Payer Claims

Database for a whole host of policy reasons. And they've been able to interject and produce reports, annual reports on spending, annual reports on the drivers of costs, but also interject in a number of different places where, where that information would not have otherwise been available to inform policy decisions, but also to inform patients in that case.

So I think there are consumer-facing things that are very useful, although I do agree that some of the private initiatives from insurers are better. But I do think that having the Health Policy Commission there to really analyze that data has been a very useful step as well.

Ms. CLARKE. Thank you. I yield back.

Mr. HARPER. The gentlewoman yields back.

The chair will now recognize the gentleman from Texas, Dr. Burgess, for 5 minutes.

Mr. BURGESS. Thank you, Mr. Chairman. And I have got way more questions than I can package into 5 minutes, but we will do our best. And I may submit some for the record.

I do appreciate both of you being here today. Let me just ask you a question, Dr. Chernew, since you brought up about the private sector initiatives versus the All Payer Claims Databases.

I pointed out in my opening statement, Texas has Texas PricePoint. I believe it is Texas Hospital Association that has done that. So, good on them for having done that. But is that not helpful for them to have done it? Does that delay getting an All Payer Claims Database set up in the state? What are some of the tensions there?

Mr. CHERNEW. I think it is at the end of the day probably marginally helpful as opposed to not. I don't think it delays All Payer Claims Databases.

I think because all healthcare is local and the states are going to do different things, I'm sort of a state experimentation kind of person in this space. I wish I could tell you I knew what would work. I don't like sounding as skeptical as I am. So I think the more we can allow states to do different things and then study what they're doing, I think the better.

Mr. BURGESS. And, Dr. King, do you have any thoughts on that? Ms. KING. I tend to agree. I think that on balance it's probably helpful. I think any attempts to provide transparency are generally useful. I don't think it probably delayed an All Payer Claims Database unless you were considering that as the alternative option and went with this one.

I think that an All Payer Claims—so, in terms of the private entity tools, I think those tend to be much more useful for consumers. Right? And so, United Healthcare they go in, you type in your name, you get into the system, and it tells you what your actual, where you are in your deductible, what your copay would be for different people.

And I think All Payer Claims Databases allow you to use the information for a lot of different purposes; right? So that's sort of the difference. One is very targeted at individuals, but you also have to be in the plan in order to see that information.

Mr. BURGESS. Sure.

Ms. KING. Right? You can't get that information when you're choosing your plan. Although Massachusetts I think just has a law coming down that would enable that, for you to see different prices as though you were in different plans.

Mr. BURGESS. Txpricepoint.org you would not have to be in a plan. That is a ——

Ms. KING. No. But it tells you——

Mr. BURGESS [continuing]. Public hospital provides database.

Ms. KING. But it doesn't tell you the price that you would pay for your insurer.

Mr. BURGESS. No, it does not.

Ms. KING. Right. So that is very hard to know what to do with those prices.

Mr. BURGESS. So, every time I see that TrueCar ad on T.V. I wonder why we don't have TrueCar for healthcare. But then as someone who had a health savings and account for years and year and always has paid the highest out-of-pocket costs for everything, hospital labs included, I was a big believer when I first heard about Theranos. And I thought, oh man, a cheap way to get a bunch of blood tests done. I'm all in. Except the reliability suffers.

Ms. KING. Yes.

Mr. BURGESS. So there is a caveat there, I guess. Is that the correct observation?

Mr. CHERNEW. Yes. And remember, it's TrueCar, it's not TrueCarborator; right? And it's TrueCar.

Mr. BURGESS. So, I think, Dr. Chernew, I think you mentioned the alternative payment methods. And going back to when the Secretary of Labor was Secretary of Health and Human Services he did a demonstration project, a physician group practice demonstration project where they dealt with some alternative payment mechanisms. I think, if I understand the history correctly, ACOs kind of grew out from there.

But can you speak to that? Is there a way to foster the development of what perhaps Secretary Leavitt's original idea was there?

Mr. CHERNEW. Yes. And I think, again maybe a little far afield, Medicare has been very innovative in the whole range of payment models. But I also can't tell you what the right type of payment models are. But I think——

Mr. BURGESS. Neither can we. But we are learning, I hope.

Mr. CHERNEW. There you go. But the more we support alternative payment models, in many ways the better.

One thing that I think does matter is to understand that the price from the point of view from the physician is different than the price from the point of view of the patient because the patient is buying some episode of care. The physician is delivering a small part of that, the same with the facilities.

So, the more for example supporting bundled payments, which Medicare is doing, the more you can support that type of thing, and the more payment moves towards more consumer-oriented sets of things that are being purchased, the closer you get to transparency because then someone will know what does it cost for a colonoscopy, not what does it cost for the technical component, the professional component, the anesthesia component, et cetera, et cetera.

Mr. BURGESS. But people still buy on provider as well as on price. Which just brings me to the final thought, and I will close my section out.

In the lead-up to the Affordable Care Act there was a lot of concern about physician-owned hospitals. And in fact, remember, physician-owned hospitals got whacked in the Affordable Care Act. Mr. Chairman, I am going to ask unanimous consent to insert a letter or a article into the record about physician behavior with physician-owned facilities.

Back in my world it was all about time. I got paid the same amount, regardless whether the patient went to an ambulatory surgery center or to a community hospital. The lab processing from my reimbursement's perspective was identical. But the cost to the patients was a fixed rate in an ambulatory surgery center, and the sky's the limit in the community hospital. I am oversimplifying.

But nevertheless, that is I think one of the pressures that we are going to have to consider as we work through these.

But, again, I ask unanimous consent to put this article into the record.

Mr. HARPER. Without objection.

[The information appears at the conclusion of the hearing.]

Mr. HARPER. The gentleman yields back.

The chair now recognize——

Mr. BURGESS. I want the gentlelady from Colorado to read it before she accepts. I thought I had found a way to get you to read my articles.

Ms. DEGETTE. I will take your word.

Mr. BURGESS. All right. Thank you, Mr. Chairman, I yield back.

Mr. HARPER. And that was on the record by the way.

And the chair will now recognize——

Ms. DEGETTE. But not under oath.

Mr. HARPER. Not under oath.

But the chair will now recognize the gentleman from California, Mr. Ruiz, for 5 minutes.

Mr. RUIZ. Thank you, Mr. Chairman.

Overall we know transparency is a good thing and leads to better understandings of market dynamics and better ways to help everybody come up with good policy that is going to really lead to a more cost-efficient way of providing better healthcare for the American people.

However, there are certain things that transparency is good for and the market really focuses on.

Like, for example, if you had the ability to make the choice, and knowledge to know the difference between the products in a situation where you can actually make a decision, and not under duress, or when you are in a coma, or when you are in cardiac arrest or something going into the emergency department, and there are some things that transparency obviously can work.

So, in your statement, however, Dr. Chernew, you note in your testimony that "many studies, including several of my own and those of my colleagues, find that transparency has minimal, if any, impact on the market." You go on to explain why transparency results in only minimal impact on price.

Dr. Chernew, it sounds like the bottom line is that it is somewhat folly to rely upon transparency as the magic bullet to bring down healthcare costs. Is that correct?

Mr. CHERNEW. Yes.

Mr. RUIZ. OK. In what situation does transparency work?

Mr. CHERNEW. When there's more commodity type services, when they're not as connected to things and you have time to shop I think transparency works.

I think independent of shopping, transparency works just to tell people what they would have to pay out of pocket. Just knowing. So, you're not going to shop, it's just you don't want to get a bill after the fact that's way higher than you thought.

So, I think transparency is useful. I think it needs to be coupled with other things.

Mr. RUIZ. But you are saying it is not what we should be focusing on?

Mr. CHERNEW. I think there's a lot of reasons why healthcare markets don't function well. Transparency I would put down on my list for what that's true.

I think it's important, let me say, what I worry about, for example, is insurance inherently, unlike most products is a pooled product. I'm in with a lot of other people on the same plan. I worry that if we allow the benefit packages to deteriorate to the point where people are paying a lot out of pocket and we separate that market through a range of things that are going on that I won't mention—it might be too partisan, I don't mean it to be—that people have higher out-of-pocket bills because they won't understand when they bought the insurance plan what was covered. They'll go to the doctor and they'll realize that what they thought was insurance wasn't that good. And it's very hard to make that work well.

Mr. RUIZ. So, do you think that putting too much weight on transparency to reduce healthcare costs is a distraction?

Mr. CHERNEW. I worry that that's the case.

Mr. RUIZ. OK. I am a doctor. And I know that patients rely on doctors' knowledge, and training, and years of experience to make decisions that will be to the best benefit for the patients. And I know that it is difficult for patients to then, if an orthopedic surgeon says I recommend a titanium type of metal for your knee replacement, that a patient in general is not going to do the research or have the know-how in order to determine what kind of equipment they want for their knee to make that best judgment.

But I do think that there is some value in transparency. I think it is just what Dr. Burgess said earlier, it is insane that one hospital will charge, I don't know, I'm just making these numbers up, but $2,000 for a colonoscopy. And then, like, across the city in the same, same region another hospital charges $10,000. So why is that?

And we should understand where are the mechanics that go into that so that we can identify, in those cases when you do have the time to choose which studies or which equipment you want where you can have the knowledge and have the time, and under the situation, to make that possible, I think we should focus on that.

But, Dr. Chernew, you also mentioned that if the objective is to meaningfully reduce healthcare costs, other strategies such as addressing adverse selection in the individual market for healthcare may be more fruitful. Can you expand on that?

So, if the objective is to lower costs are there ways to combine transparency initiative with some of these other efforts to lower costs? Can you go into that?

Mr. CHERNEW. Well, let me talk about two separate things very quickly. The first one is transparency is important to support almost all of the various new benefit design things we do. It's important for a range of public regulation things. I think there's a bunch of reasons why transparency matters. And I think it's unconscionable, some of the stories that I'm sure your constituents have told you. I think that's a really big deal.

That said, the biggest problems we have in a lot of healthcare markets aren't related to transparency, they're related to how we hold the market together and how the benefit design packages play out. So, at Harvard we control exactly the benefit package. We push everybody into it. It's pooled, it works.

If you allow markets to spin out of control and let people do various things there's implications of that that differ from markets for cars, or markets for asparagus, or things like that. So, figuring out how to address those types of problems so you don't have individuals that end up in insurance plans where they're going to be charged a lot out of pocket I think are important.

Mr. RUIZ. Harvard. Harvard Business School?

Mr. CHERNEW. Harvard University. Harvard University has a Benefits Committee that offers benefits for all of the schools.

Mr. RUIZ. OK.

Mr. CHERNEW. So, Business, the Medical School, the main part.

And we advise the Provost, for the non-union workers, about how to deal with our challenges. And we have a lot of challenges.

Mr. HARPER. The gentleman yields back.

The chair will now recognize the gentlewoman from Indiana, the chair of our Ethics Committee, Ms. Brooks, for 5 minutes.

Mrs. BROOKS. Thank you, Mr. Chairman.

And I want to stay on that line of questioning, Dr. Chernew.

Speaking of employers, and you mentioned Harvard specifically, and even some insurers provide transparency tools to their members or their employees, and have redesigned plans and networks to encourage price shopping, can you describe some of the features of the price transparency tools that are adopted by employers and insurers, whether it is Harvard or others, and how they differ from the state transparency initiatives?

Mr. CHERNEW. Yes. So, and again Dr. King mentioned, if you are in a plan that offers one of these types of transparency tools and you know you need a service, you can go in and type the service. Now, that actually sounds easy. But remember, if you're shopping for a CT scan, there's 50 types of CT scans, and it depends on what the dyes are, so it's not as easy as you think.

It will aggregate out and try and come up with a number. It will combine the physician and the hospital. Because you don't care how much is going to the hospital and how much is going to the physician, you care totally what are you going to pay——

Mrs. BROOKS. Right.

Mr. CHERNEW [continuing]. For the whole thing. It will know, and again it won't know perfectly because there's time lags, it will know within reason where you are in your deductible. So, if you are over the top of your deductible it will give you a different price quote than if you haven't yet spent your deductible.

Most of the public non-insurer-based tools don't have all that information, so they cannot tell you very accurately what you would pay. They don't. We know what prices our carriers have negotiated with all the different providers. But most public tools don't know— New Hampshire being an exception—the prices that different providers have negotiated with different insurers. And they certainly don't know where you are in terms of your deductible.

Mrs. BROOKS. And do you, are you familiar with a lot of private tools like what you have just described, and are these types of tools, whether they are insurers or employers, are they proving to be effective in changing consumer behavior——

Mr. CHERNEW. So, the tools——

Mrs. BROOKS [continuing]. And reducing steps?

Mr. CHERNEW [continuing]. Are almost always tools that employers offer but the insurers make. The employers don't do much. They buy things. So, the insurers are the ones that offer the tools. Or other, there's a firm Castlight, for example, that's well known for having these types of tools and selling to employers who can buy access to them. And they have been, unfortunately, disappointingly ineffective.

Mrs. BROOKS. Why, do you believe?

Mr. CHERNEW. Well, for one, even the best of them are very complicated. The people care more about their physician than the tool, so they're hesitant to shop. And in many cases the employers have provided the transparency tools but haven't designed their benefit packages in ways that make them really salient. So you get back the same result.

Even if there—you've mentioned, several people have mentioned that there's wide variation in prices across markets, $2,000 and $500. But most patients don't pay $2,000 and $500 to their employers, most of them only pay—if you were at Harvard you'd pay $30 flat fee no matter where you went to. So the tool doesn't help you that much.

Mrs. BROOKS. Dr. King, would you like to comment on the private initiatives, private, the private tools?

Ms. KING. Yes. So I would just basically reiterate what Dr. Chernew said, that they haven't seen the kinds of results that they would be looking for. And I know that Castlight has been, is employers basically buy Castlight Health and offer it to their employees. And they found very low engagement from employees.

I think a lot of employees don't want to shop for providers. They don't necessarily want to shop. They will shop a little bit for the shoppable services. But they haven't seen the overall level of engagement has been about 3 to 6 percent on a lot of those tools.

Mrs. BROOKS. Well, and I would like to ask both of you why do you believe that is the case? Why is it that we have these tools, whether it is a private sector, an employer, or at the state base that states have invested in these, why do we have such low engagement on this issue?

Ms. KING. I think that we largely have low engagement, partly because people aren't incentivized to use them. If you pay the same price you're not that much incentivized to use them. But I also think it goes back to this idea that when you go to your provider and they make a recommendation for you of which provider to go to for your hip surgery, or which lab to go to. Oh, go to the lab down the street. It's unlikely to then, to whip out your laptop and figure out if there's a cheaper provider elsewhere.

Also, a lot of times individual providers prefer that their patients use a particular lab——

Mrs. BROOKS. Right.

Ms. KING [continuing]. Because they know that they get the results quickly, or it goes right into their EMR, or there are some synergies within the system.

And so I think that patients are reluctant to go against their provider's advice or recommendation, which is why you should try to get this information into the hands of the providers so that if they think I would recommend five doctors to do your hip surgery. Oh, two of them are in your network. Let's talk about you'd pay $500 for this doctor, and you'd pay $200 for this doctor, let's talk about the benefits and detriments of that. That's what we need.

Mrs. BROOKS. And, Dr. Chernew, anything different on that as to why we have such low rate of use?

Mr. CHERNEW. Yes. I think that it is a mistake to believe that consumers fundamentally want to shop. They actually fundamentally want to pay less out of pocket, and they want things to be simpler. That's what they really want because of all these sort of interactions with their physicians.

And so they tend not to want to go find these things out. You can push at the margins, but as a main view that we're going to use market forces to fundamentally control our problems I think is a little optimistic, as much as that pains me to say as an economist.

Mrs. BROOKS. Thank you both. I yield back. Mr. HARPER. The gentlewoman yields back.

The chair will now recognize the gentleman from New York, Mr. Tonko, for 5 minutes.

Mr. TONKO. Thank you, Mr. Chair. And welcome to our guests. Many states and healthcare systems have implemented a variety of programs that are intended to give consumers additional information about the price of healthcare services on the theory that this will allow consumers to make more informed decisions and perhaps lower their costs. They are listening to your concerns there.

But maybe you can develop for us a little better some of the tools and some of the concerns that we should have.

Academics, including both of you today, have studied these reforms to see what works, what doesn't work, and where we might go from here. I would like to spend a few minutes discussing with our panelists what the academic literature has to say about these efforts.

Dr. Chernew, in your written testimony you use the example of shopping for a car to describe why transparency doesn't always work to bring down the cost of shopping for healthcare and the like. Could you briefly describe what makes shopping for healthcare different and more complicated than that which we would utilize for products or services?

Mr. CHERNEW. Most products or services are bundled in a way that you care about. So you're not buying the ingredients. When you go buy a meal you don't price out all the individual ingredients, it all comes together.

Healthcare, because of the history of the way in which it developed, and because the reimbursement system was really provider focused so you, remember, physicians and hospitals, they're inputs to providing care. Right? But you really care about the joint product. And so that has made it difficult to simply give prices that have been developed from sort of a payer perspective to consumers who are purchasing from a different perspective. And it, broadly speaking, has been hard for people to shop in that way. Combine that with insurance distorting prices, the reliance on physicians, the complexity of the problem, the salience of the problem altogether has made it very hard for people to shop.

Mr. TONKO. And, also, you wrote in an August 2017 "Health Affairs" article that "simply offering a transparency tool is not sufficient to meaningfully decrease healthcare prices or spending."

So, what did you find regarding these transparency tools? And why were they unable to bring down the prices on their own?

Mr. CHERNEW. They're often offered with the narrative of they're going to help make markets work. And because most people don't use them, because they're complicated, they don't make markets work that well on their own, and as a result you don't see prices respond.

Mr. TONKO. So, could you describe what conditions would be sufficient to meaningfully bring these costs down?

Mr. CHERNEW. Well, there's bringing costs overall down is challenging. What's sufficient to how transparency tools work, which I believe are true in a limited number of cases, is you need to have services bundled in a way that people can understand. You need to have benefit designs done in a way that make people actually feel the cost at the margin. And you need to avoid a situation in which the physicians that are making the recommendations are, for example, owned by a system, so the physician's going to refer within a system. And once you choose your primary care doctor you're actually choosing a whole referral network they use, and it's very hard to get them to work.

So, I think Dr. King and I agree that the margins is all valuable. There are specific cases. It's really valuable to let people know what they might have to pay out of pocket. But as a fundamental question about what could you all do to all of a sudden use transparency to revolutionize the way that consumers shop, and therefore to control healthcare spending, that's a really tall order.

Mr. TONKO. Thank you.

And, Dr. King, your written testimony discusses the usefulness of state efforts such as All Payer Claims Databases to bring down prices for consumers. These databases are intended to house a comprehensive collection of medical claims data from both public and private payers on how much they pay for different kinds of procedures.

How can consumers use that information in these databases to inform their healthcare decisions? And what are the limitations on this kind of data?

Ms. KING. Thank you. So, basically the consumers wouldn't use the database themselves. The information that's housed in the database would then have to get put into a consumer-facing website like what New Hampshire has on Health Costs. And that has been demonstrated to bring down costs a little bit and allow patients to use it.

So if you have the negotiated rate between a provider and an insurance company in all of these All Payer Claims Databases, and all of the utility, how we utilize healthcare, who patients go to, what they charge, what the negotiated rates are across the State, you could then generate really meaningful information for patients because you would know which insurance company they were in and what that insurance company had negotiated its prices with providers for. And you could use that to populate consumer-facing websites and consumer-facing tools that would provide patients with information on their out-of-pocket costs.

I just want to say that one of the other things that we haven't really discussed today as a driver of costs that affects transparency is the fact that a huge majority of our markets for healthcare are highly concentrated. And one of the reasons why we have such a problem with transparency is that you have provider organizations and provider systems with a large amount of market power and they can demand to keep their prices secret. They can negotiate things in ways that drive up costs and then, and then hinder transparency to find that out.

And so, if you were really looking, I think transparency is important at the margins. I think it's useful. I think it's generally a good thing in a capitalist society for people to know what they're going to pay. But I also think if we want to talk about competition and why the markets don't work you need to look at the markets themselves and figure out that competition is dwindling and dying because these markets are so consolidated.

Mr. TONKO. Thank you very much. And, Mr. Chair, I yield back my time.

Mr. HARPER. The gentleman yields back.

And the chair will now recognize the gentleman from Georgia, Mr. Carter, for 5 minutes.

Mr. CARTER. Thank you, Mr. Chairman. And thank both of you for being here.

Dr. King, I am going to let you continue on because you have hit on the right point, the vertical integration that we are experiencing right now. What you have is you have a PBM who owns a pharmacy. Now the PBM and the pharmacy are talking about buying an insurance company. Now you have got an insurance company, Cigna, talking about buying the PBM, which also owns the pharmacies.

The vertical integration and lack of competition is something. And then they can hide it all throughout that vertical integration. They don't care where they make it, as long as they make it. But that is the problem. You hit the nail on the head right there.

Anything else you want to add to that?

Ms. KING. I just want, I just want to pile on. So, I ——

Mr. CARTER. Sure.

Ms. KING. I think that in some instances we're seeing integration and it's not just vertical; right? We're seeing horizontal integration.

We're seeing vertical integration. And now we're also starting to see cross-market integration where hospitals are buying provider systems in other parts of the state, other, and in other states. And the more integrated these markets become overall, the less competition we are able to have.

Mr. CARTER. And that is the whole key. Transparency is eminently important, no question about it. But competition is the key as well. And being able to see that competition, we have used the example about buying a car. I believe it is New Hampshire who has a database, a website you can go to to compare medical costs. That is the kind of thing we are talking about, and that is what is going to lead to decreasing healthcare costs.

Ms. KING. Well, that's right. And if there's very little competition in the state, or you have an entity with an extreme amount of market power, they are able to keep prices very high, regardless of how transparent you make them.

Mr. CARTER. Right.

Ms. KING. If you don't have a choice of where to go, they can charge you whatever they want.

Mr. CARTER. OK. Let me get to my part. First of all, Mr. Chairman, I want to ask unanimous consent to submit two letters, one from the National Community Pharmacists Association and another from the American Pharmacists Association for the record.

Mr. HARPER. Without objection, so ordered.

[The information appears at the conclusion of the hearing.]

Mr. CARTER. Thank you very much.

I need to get back very quickly to a question that Representative Barton asked about the coupons being used in Medicare Part D. The anti-kickback, as you know, that will prohibit that from happening. But one thing my colleagues need to keep in mind is that a lot, most of these coupons are for brand name drugs. And if you get outside of that formulary it is going to end up costing taxpayer more.

And every quickly, the reason that happens is because when a patient goes and meets their deductible, then goes into the donut, if they increase the costs by buying the ones that are off the formulary then they get into the catastrophic quickly, more quickly, which means that the taxpayers are going to be paying more for their insurance, for that patient's insurance. It is going to end up actually costing taxpayers more.

So that is one of the reasons why the Medicare Part D CMS does not allow that to happen in there. So I want to make sure we got that clear.

Representative Griffith mentioned my legislation dealing with gag clauses. Twenty-two states have implemented this thus far. We need to implement it at the Federal level. Here we are in America with freedom of speech, and over 30 years of experience in working in pharmacy and I could never tell a patient, look, if you pay for this out of your pocket it will only cost you $7.00, but your copay is going to be $20.00. And that is just ridiculous for us, particularly here in America, not to be able to do that.

I wanted to talk also about PBMs and their licensure and registration. A number of states have required PBMs to register with their insurance commissions. And the most recent one was Arkansas held a special session. And now they have enacted the Arkansas Pharmacy Benefit

Licensure Act where the state insurance department requires PBMs to license within the state.

One of the things, also, we talk about pharmacies. The number one pharmacy in America, CVS, they have more stores. Walgreens. You know what number three is? Express Scripts with their mail order pharmacies. Yet, they do not have to register in each state.

Don't you think they should at least have to register in each state, the third largest pharmacy chain in America? And they are nothing but mail order pharmacies. Surely they should have to register in every state.

Any comment.

Ms. KING. I know very little about it but it sounds like you're right, yes.

Mr. CARTER. OK. I know.

So, anyway, Dr. King, Medicaid managed care organizations, that is another way that we can attack some of these costs as well because without having, without having the transparency there to see what exactly the PBMs are charging in those, then we are unable to control costs.

In fact, West Virginia just did away with their managed—they carved that out and saved $30 million. In Ohio they saved $227 million. In Kentucky they figured their costs would be $380 million. Why can't we control that on a Federal level as well?

We have a number of managed care organization contracts at the Federal level. If we could control those, do you think we could have—and had transparency in it, do you think we could save costs there?

We could. The answer is yes. I'm sorry. Mr. HARPER. The gentleman yields back.

The chair will now recognize the gentlewoman from Illinois, Ms. Schakowsky, for 5 minutes.

Ms. SCHAKOWSKY. Thank you.

Dr. Chernew, I have never heard a witness, though I am sure many are thinking of it, that I wish my time were over. And I have been chuckling over that for most of the hearing.

You mentioned the idea that pharmaceutical companies, manufacturers can charge whatever the market will bear. But the question is, what is the market?

We have a briefing from a Dr. Anderson from Hopkins who said, for example, Sovaldi, that they decided that all they really needed to make back the money that they invested in Sovaldi, or the marketing that they do, they need 20 percent of the market.

So, we are not talking about widgets, we are not talking about cars, we are talking about illness, life, death. And so if they charge, which they did, $86,000 for this cure to Hep C, all they really care about is that if 20 percent of people who have this really awful disease can get cured.

And so it seems to me that we ought to have a better way. When you say charge whatever they want to make the money they want, this isn't about free markets, this is about a very segmented market. I just wonder if you would comment on that?

Mr. CHERNEW. I wrote in my written testimony that I was going to avoid pharmaceutical markets because it raises so many complicated issues. But since asked, I will dip my toe in.

The challenge, and I will use Sovaldi as an example, is Sovaldi was a truly innovative drug. And all analyses suggest at least most any value criteria you would have. And although it may be difficult for people to swallow—that's not a pill joke—but anyway, it turns out that the evidence suggests that with greater incentives for prescription drug innovation you get more innovation.

The problem is that statement should not imply that the drug companies get a blank check. And therein lies the basic problem.

I do not think their goal was simply to make back their R&D money. Their goal was to make more money.

Ms. SCHAKOWSKY. Yes.

Mr. CHERNEW. Right? That's the goal in capitalist societies, to make more money. And in fact they have created a remarkably good product that for decades will benefit us and everybody. Right?

Ms. SCHAKOWSKY. Not everybody.

Mr. CHERNEW. The challenge——

Ms. SCHAKOWSKY. The people who can pay for it.

Mr. CHERNEW. No, that's right. So the people who can't pay for it and don't get it, they're in the same place off they were before it got invented. So, the challenge is how to manage the incentives for innovation, which are really important, with the obvious egregious problems of pricing. Not simply for what people who pay out of pocket. It's the out-of-pocket comments that bring everybody here. But the charge, to deal with the overall total amount of spending, and the prices, and the volume for all of these drugs.

Ms. SCHAKOWSKY. You know what, let me stop because I have one more——

Mr. CHERNEW. Thank you.

Ms. SCHAKOWSKY [continuing]. One more question about it.

But I think it is worse if you know that there is the cure right there, that there is a cure right there and you can't get it. I think in some ways it is worse than thinking there isn't one.

But, again, about—OK, so you don't want to talk about markets, but I just want to mention this. One argument is that increased competition or more generic drugs are going to lead to lower drug prices. But recently Elizabeth Rosenthal described the bizarre phenomenon economists call sticky pricing where prices of competing prescription drugs simply rise together with each new drug that is provided.

So, we have got Novartis, a cancer drug. And Gleevec was first listed at $26,000 in the market. And the first generic was list priced at around $140,000 annually. And now many drugs in the same family as Gleevec cost on average $150,000 per year.

So, we aren't seeing. Again, markets in drugs, very different. We are seeing an increase. So, this thought that competition is going to drive it down and generics will drive it down, not working always.

Mr. CHERNEW. Always. I agree.

So, if you look at drugs at 15 years ago we could have been arguing about Lipitor and a whole series of other blockbuster drugs. They've all gone generic. We buy them at Harvard, they're bought as generic. It's a great deal. And there's a lot of real advances.

The challenges that are presented through some of those drugs, through biosimilars, which is a whole different issue, becomes important, are really, really, really important. And the issues you're raising I'm incredibly sympathetic with because the basic problem is we've been very successful at encouraging amazing innovation.

We haven't found a good way to make sure that that innovation is affordable for people. And even if you solve the problem that people are paying a lot out of pocket, the prices getting passed through through insurance premiums create a really fundamental challenge.

Ms. SCHAKOWSKY. OK, but I just want—and I know my time is up—but we are seeing increases in drugs that have been on the market for decades. They charge what the market will bear, and that means that the prices have kept going up out of control.

So, I can't let you answer. I am sorry, I am out of time. And you should be happy.

Mr. HARPER. The gentlewoman yields back.

The chair will now recognize the gentleman from Pennsylvania, Mr. Costello, for 5 minutes.

Mr. COSTELLO. Thank you, Mr. Chairman.

Dr. Chernew, in your written testimony you noted that one of the many reasons that many transparency initiatives have had only a minimal impact on the market is because consolidation in the healthcare markets limits choice. Consolidation in the healthcare industry is something that is of great interest to this committee. As Chairman Harper mentioned at the beginning of the hearing, the O&I Subcommittee had a hearing on consolidation in the healthcare market last February.

Do you think that there has been too much consolidation in the healthcare market? And, if so, what impact has it had on healthcare costs?

Second piece of the question, how does consolidation limit the effectiveness of both private and public transparency initiatives?

Mr. CHERNEW. Yes, there's too much consolidation and it's raised the prices and spending.

And the consolidation makes it difficult for transparency initiatives to work because they fundamentally require choice. If there's no choice, knowing the price of an office charge doesn't help you all that much.

The only thing I will say is don't think about transparency as only working through consumers. Having the regulators, having the policy commission, having journalists see the prices can also be helpful. But by and large the more consolidation, the harder it is to get markets to work and, therefore, the harder it is to get transparency to work.

Mr. COSTELLO. I have a question for you. But would you like anything to add, Dr. King? You were shaking your head yes before.

Ms. KING. Yes. Well, I'm in vehement agreement with most of the things he has said today.

So, I think that also transparency can help with the consolidation problem because you can actually, if you have a good All Payer Claims Database you can look and see how a particular merger or acquisition over time drove up costs or didn't drive up costs.

Did they actually gain the efficiencies they said they were going to get when they actually merged?

Did they pass it through to consumers? You'd be able to know that. And you'd be able to then turn around and stop future consolidation in the markets through that.

So, I think that those work both ways.

Mr. COSTELLO. Dr. King, thank you. In your written testimony you highlighted how states could use healthcare claims data reported to an APCD to examine the drivers of healthcare costs over time, the impact of mergers, acquisitions, and other affiliations on healthcare price and quality, among other things, similar to what you just were sharing with us right there.

How would the healthcare claims data reported to an APCD give states with an APCD unique insight into the impact of M&As that states without an APCD would not have?

Ms. KING. So, currently because a lot of these private prices are shrouded in secrecy, the attorney general doesn't know and other state entities don't actually have the data to examine how mergers in the past have affected prices, or they don't have the ability to project how mergers in the future might affect prices.

And so, if you have this enormous database of healthcare prices over time that allows you to look at utilization patterns, how people went, were funneled to different providers, and the cost, you could then make much better economic projections about how a merger might affect things in the future. And, also, you'd be able to look back in the past and see if they kept their promise.

Mr. COSTELLO. Can you describe the general approaches states have been taking regarding the pharmaceutical price transparency bills you have seen?

Ms. KING. Yes. So, states have looked at a number of different things with regard to price to pharmaceuticals this year. This has been the big topic among the states. They have done everything from a lot of price, pharmaceutical price disclosure anti-gag clauses this year.

They have also looked at pricing reports or requiring pharmaceutical companies to submit reports at the end of the year, annually or at some other time that basically describe how much it cost them to produce a drug, what they spent on development and marketing, and then what, how they're pricing their drugs, both as an annual cost, as an individual patient cost.

States have also focused on gag prohibitions and disclosures, pricing reports. And that's a lot of what we've seen with respect to pharmaceuticals. And then a lot of PBM regulation as well, trying to promote transparency amongst the pharmacy benefit managers.

Mr. COSTELLO. Thank you. I will yield back. Mr. HARPER. The gentleman yields back.

I want to thank both of you for being here today, giving us some very valuable insight and information as we tackle this very important challenge that we have.

So, I want to thank the members that have participated in today's hearing. And I will remind members that they have 10 business days to submit questions for the record. And should you receive any written questions, we would ask the witnesses to respond as quickly as possible to those questions.

The subcommittee is adjourned.

[Whereupon, at 12:02 p.m., the subcommittee was adjourned.]

[Material submitted for inclusion in the record follows:]

U.S. HOUSE OF REPRESENTATIVES COMMITTEE ON ENERGY AND COMMERCE

July 15, 2018

TO: Members, Subcommittee on Oversight and Investigations

FROM: Committee Majority Staff

RE: Hearing entitled "Examining State Efforts to Improve Transparency of Health Care Costs for Consumers."

The Subcommittee on Oversight and Investigations will hold a hearing on Tuesday, July 17, 2018, at 10:15 a.m. in 2322 Rayburn House Office Building, entitled "Examining State Efforts to Improve Transparency of Health Care Costs for Consumers." The purpose of the hearing is to examine state laws and policies that improve transparency of health care costs for consumers and the impact that they had on consumers.

I. Witnesses

- Jaime King, Professor, UC Hastings College of the Law, Associate Dean and Co- Director, UCSF/UC Hastings Consortium on Law, Science, and Health Policy;
- Michael Chernew, Leonard D. Schaeffer Professor of Health Care Policy, Director, Healthcare Markets and Regulation Lab, Department of Health Care Policy, Harvard Medical School; and

- Kavita Patel, Associate ChicfMedical Officer, Johns Hopkins Medicine.

II. Background

A. Health Care Expenditures

In 2016, U.S health care spending was estimated to be about $3.3 trillion, and the overall share of gross domestic product (GDP) related to health care spending was 17.9 percent (up from percent in 2015).[102] According to the Centers for Medicare and Medicaid Services (CMS), 32 percent of the $3.3 trillion in expenditures was spent on hospital care, 20 percent was spent on physician and clinical services, 14 percent was spent on other (including, but not limited to home health care and durable medical equipment), 10 percent was spent on prescription drugs, 8 percent was spent on government administration and net cost of health insurance, 5 percent was spent on nursing care facilities and continuing care retirement communities, 5 percent was spent on investment, and 4 percent was spent on dental services.[103] The majority—75 percent—of the $3.3 trillion in expenditures was paid for by health insurance (34 percent by private health insurance, 20 percent by Medicare, 17 percent by Medicaid, and 4 percent by the U.S. Department of Veterans Affairs (VA), the U.S. Department of Defense (DOD), and the Children's Health Insurance Program (CHIP)).[104]

According to a Kaiser Family Foundation analysis of National Health Expenditure data released by CMS, total health expenditures have

[102] U.S. Dep't of Health and Human Services, Centers for Medicare & Medicaid Services, *National Health Expenditures 2016 Highlights* (Dec. 2017), *available at* https://www.cms.gov/Research-Statistics-Data-and-Systems/Statistics-Trends-and-Reports/NationalHealthExpendData/Downloads/highlights.pdf.

[103] U.S. Dep't of Health and Human Services, Centers for Medicare & Medicaid Services, *The Nation's Health Dollar ($3.3 Trillion), Calendar Year 2016: Where it Came From, Where it Went* (Dec. 2017), *available at* https://www.cms.gov/Research-Statistics-Data-and-Systems/Statistics-Trends-and-Reports/NationalHealthExpendData/Downloads/PieChart SourcesExpenditures.pdf.

[104] *Id.*

increased substantially over the past several decades.[105] Indeed, data released by CMS indicates that total health expenditures in the U.S. were about $721 billion in 1990, $1.4 trillion in 2000, $2.4 trillion in 2008, and $3.3 trillion in 2016.[106] Moreover, on a per capita basis, health spending has also grown—increasing from $8,412 in 2010 to $10,348 in 2016.[107] Although health care expenditures have continued to increase at a rapid pace, U.S. health care spending increased in 2016 at a slower rate than in previous years (in 2016, spending on health care increased by 4.3 percent compared to 5.1 percent in 2014 and 5.8 percent in 2015).[108]

Many different factors may influence health care spending, including, but not limited to, population aging, prices, policy changes, consolidation, and public and private initiatives.[109] Moreover, some research has shown that there may be significant variation in the cost of health care services in one geographic region, and that more expensive health care services are not always associated with a higher quality of care.[110] For example, a 2014 study by the U.S. Government Accountability Office (GAO), found that "the estimated total cost of maternity care at selected acute care hospitals in the Boston area that rated more highly on several quality indicators ranged between $6,834 and $21,554 (consumers would pay between

---

[105] Rabah Kamal and Cynthia Cox, Peterson-Kaiser Health System Tracker, *How has U.S. spending on health care changed over time?* (Dec. 20, 2017), *available at* https://www.healthsystemtracker.org/chart-collection/u-s-spending-healthcare-changed-time/#item-total-health-expenditures-increased-substantially-past-several- decades_2017.

[106] *Id.*

[107] *Id.*

[108] Micah Hartman, et al., *National Health Care Spending in 2016: Spending and Enrollment Growth Slow After Initial Coverage Expansions*, HEALTH AFFAIRS, Vol. 37, No. 1 (Dec. 6, 2017), *available at* https://www.healthaffairs.org/doi/full/10.1377/hlthaff.2017.1299.

[109] Aaron C. Catlin and Cathy A. Cowan, *History of Health Spending in the United States, 1960-2013* (Nov. 19, 2015), *available at* https://www.cms.gov/Research-Statistics-Data-and-Systems/Statistics-Trends-and-Reports/NationalHealthExpendData/Downloads/HistoricalNHEPaper.pdf; Sean P. Keehan, et al., *National Health Expenditure Projections, 2016-25: Price Increases, Aging Push Sector to 20 Percent of Economy*, HEALTH AFFAIRS (Mar. 2017), *available at* https://www.ssc.wisc.edu/~gwallace/Papers/Health%20Aff-2017-Keehan-hlthaff.2016.1627%20(1).pdf; Medicare Payment Advisory Commission (MedPAC), *Report to the Congress: Medicare and the Health Care Delivery System, Chapter 10: Provider Consolidation: The Role of Medicare Policy* (June 2017).

[110] U.S. Government Accountability Office (GAO), *Health Care Transparency: Actions Needed to Improve Cost and Quality Information for Consumers*, GAO-15-11, at 11 (Oct. 20, 2014).

$2,967 and $5,000 in estimated out-of-pocket costs)."[111] Similarly, in Massachusetts, the median price of magnetic resonance imaging (MRI) of the spine ranges from $500 to $1,670.[112]

Consumers are increasingly responsible for more of their health care costs. According to CMS, in 2016, consumers directly paid for about 11 percent of the $3.3 trillion spent on health care and out-of-pocket spending grew at the fastest rate of growth in 2016 since 2007.[113] In an April 2018 report, America's Health Insurance Plans (AHIP) indicated that the number of individuals enrolled in Health Savings Account (HSA)-Qualified High Deductible Health Plans (HDHPs) has been increasing, and that as of January 2017, 52 health insurance providers reported that over 21.8 million people were enrolled in an HSA-Qualified HDHP.[114] This is a significant increase over the approximately 10 million individuals enrolled in an HSA-Qualified HDHP in 2010.

B. Health Care Price Transparency Efforts

Overview

As consumers pay more for their health care, there has been an increasing amount of discussion about the role of health care price transparency for consumers and the importance of providing consumers

---

[111] *Id.* at 12.

[112] Ateev Mehrotra, M.D., M.P.H., Michael E. Chernew, Ph.D, and Anna D. Sinaiko, Ph.D., *Promise and Reality of Price Transparency*, THE NEW ENGLAND JOURNAL OF MEDICINE, at 1348 (Apr. 8, 2018); *See also* Zack Cooper, et al., *The Price Ain't Right? Hospital Prices and Health Spending on the Privately Insured*, HEALTH CARE PRICING PROJECT, at 21 (May 8, 2018), *available at* http://www.healthcarepricingproject.org/sites/default/files/20180507_variationmanuscript_0.pdf.

[113] U.S. Dep't of Health and Human Services, Centers for Medicare & Medicaid Services, *National Health Expenditures 2016 Highlights* (Dec. 2017), *available at* https://www.cms.gov/Research-Statistics-Data-and-Systems/Statistics-Trends-and-Reports/NationalHealthExpendData/Downloads/highlights.pdf; U.S. Dep't of Health and Human Services, Centers for Medicare & Medicaid Services, *The Nation's Health Dollar ($3.3 Trillion), Calendar Year 2016: Where it Came From, Where it Went* (Dec. 2017), *available at* https://www.cms.gov/Research- Statistics-Data-and -Systems/Statistics-Trends-and- Reports/NationalHealthExpendData/Downloads/PieChartSourcesExpenditures.pdf.

[114] America's Health Insurance Plans (AHIP), *Health Savings Accounts and High Deductible Health Plans Grow as Valuable Financial Planning Tools*, at 3 (Apr. 2018), *available at* https://www.ahip.org/wp- content/uploads/2018/04/HSA_Report_4.12.18.pdf.

with information that enables them to make informed health care decisions.[115] Some experts have reasoned that providing patients with information about health care costs may help reduce spending and improve care by empowering patients to make informed health care decisions.[116] Other experts, however, have questioned whether some of the current efforts to engage patients and provide them with information about the costs of health care services have successfully lowered health care expenditures and encouraged price shopping.[117] Recently, the Secretary of the Department of Health and Human Services (HHS), Alex Azar, highlighted the potential value of price transparency.[118] Azar said that "if we want to move to a system where we put patients more in charge of their own healthcare dollars, providers and insurers have to become more transparent about their pricing. There is no more powerful force than an informed consumer."[119]

Many states have taken steps to improve price transparency in the health care market and lower health care costs. These transparency efforts have generally attempted to provide consumers with information about different types of health care costs, including, but not limited to,

---

[115] *See, e.g.*, U.S. Government Accountability Office (GAO), *Health Care Transparency: Actions Needed to Improve Cost and Quality Information for Consumers*, GAO-15-11, at 1 (Oct. 20, 2014).

[116] *See, e.g.*, Robert Wood Johnson Foundation, *How Price Transparency Can Control the Cost of Health Care*, Health Policy Snapshot Series (Mar. 1, 2016), *available at* https://www.rwjf.org/en/library/research/2016/03/how- price-transparency-controls-health-care-cost.html; Health Care Cost Institute, *Issue Brief: Spending on Shoppable Services in Health Care* (Mar. 2016), *available at* http://www.healthcostinstitute.org/files/ Shoppable%20Services% 20IB%203.2.16_0.pdf; Chapin White, et al., *Policy Analysis: Healthcare Price Transparency: Policy Approaches and Estimated Impacts on Spending* (May 2014), *available at* http://www.westhealth.org/wp- content/uploads/2015/05/Price-Transparency-Policy-Analysis-FINAL-5-2-14.pdf; Bobbi Coluni, *White Paper: Save $36 Billion in U.S. Healthcare Spending Through Price Transparency*, Thomson Reuters (Feb. 2012), *available at* http://64.64.16.103/wp-content/uploads/2012/09/thomsonreuters_ savings_from_price_transparency.pdf.

[117] *See, e.g.*, Sunita Desai, et al., *Association Between Availability of a Price Transparency Tool and Outpatient Spending*, JAMA (May 3, 2016), *available at* https://jamanetwork.com/journals/jama/fullarticle/2518264.

[118] Alex M. Azar II, *Remarks on Value-Based Transformation to the Federation of American Hospitals* (Mar. 5, 2018), *available at* https://www.hhs.gov/about/leadership/ secretary/speeches/2018-speeches/remarks-on-value-based-transformation-to-the-federation-of-american-hospitals.html.

[119] *Id.*

information about the cost of health care services and/or the cost of prescription drugs. The state initiatives encouraging more transparency on prescription drug costs have taken a variety of different approaches, including, but not limited to, requiring drug manufacturers to submit information about price increases, requiring drug manufacturers to report information regarding the prices of prescription drugs and the costs associated with developing and marketing them, and prohibiting "gag clauses" that restrict pharmacists from disclosing price options to customers.[120] According to the National Conference of State Legislatures (NCSL), 22 states enacted laws between 2016 and May 31, 2018, prohibiting "gag clauses" in contracts that prohibit pharmacies from telling consumers about alternative pricing options for prescription drugs.[121]

Similarly, state efforts to promote price transparency for the cost of health care services have also have varied in approach. For instance, some state efforts have required that providers report certain pricing information to the state or the patient while other efforts have required that insurers submit certain pricing information.[122] Likewise, some state initiatives have required that pricing information be publicly posted while other initiatives have required that the information be given to the individual patient before they receive medical care.[123] Sections II.B.ii and II.B.iii of this memorandum provide a non-exhaustive list of examples of health care

---

[120] National Conference of State Legislatures, Prescription Drug Resource Center, *Recent Approaches in State Prescription Drug Laws* (Apr. 4, 2018), *available at* https://kaiserhealthnews.files.wordpress.com/2018/04/recent- approaches-in-state-prescription-drug-laws-discussion-march-2018-002.pdf; National Conference of State Legislatures, Prescription Drug Resource Center, *Prohibiting PBM "Gag Clauses" that Restrict Pharmacists from Disclosing Price Options: Recent State Legislation 2016-2018* (Jun. 1, 2018), *available at* http://www.ncsl.org/Portals/1/Documents/Health/Pharmacist_Gag_clauses-2018-14523.pdf.

[121] National Conference of State Legislatures, Prescription Drug Resource Center, *Prohibiting PBM "Gag Clauses" that Restrict Pharmacists from Disclosing Price Options: Recent State Legislation 2016-2018* (Jun. 1, 2018), *available at* http://www.ncsl.org/Portals/1/Documents/Health/Pharmacist_Gag_clauses-2018-14523.pdf.

[122] National Conference of State Legislatures, T*ransparency and Disclosure of Health Costs and Provider Statements: State Actions (*last updated Mar. 2017), *available at* http://www.ncsl.org/research/health/transparency- and-disclosure-health-costs.aspx.

[123] Ateev Mehrotra, M.D., M.P.H., Michael E. Chernew, Ph.D, and Anna D. Sinaiko, Ph.D., *Promise and Reality of Price Transparency*, THE NEW ENGLAND JOURNAL OF MEDICINE, at 1348-49 (Apr. 8, 2018).

transparency tools adopted by the states and other stakeholders that help inform patients about the costs of health care services.

As some of these transparency initiatives have been discussed and implemented, many stakeholders have highlighted the importance of considering several factors to ensure that, when a transparency tool is adopted, it conveys health care cost information to consumers in a meaningful way. For example, in 2014, the Healthcare Financial Management Association (HFMA) issued a report entitled "Price Transparency in Health Care" outlining five principles for the development of price transparency tools.[124] These principles include, among other things, that "price transparency should empower patients and other care purchasers to make meaningful price comparisons prior to receiving care," and "that price transparency should ultimately provide patients with the information they need to understand the total price of their care and what is included in that price."[125] Similarly, in an October 2014 report, GAO noted that "[t]ransparency tools are most effective if they provide information relevant to consumers and convey information in a way that consumers can readily understand" and identified 15 characteristics of effective transparency tools.[126] Moreover, one economist at the Kellogg School of Management at Northwestern University recently found that health care consumers will price shop, but only if the information is conveyed in a simple, and understandable manner.[127]

Some of the factors that make it difficult to convey price information to consumers in a meaningful way includes, but is not limited to, the fact that: (1) price information is oftentimes most useful for insured customers if it includes specific information about their particular insurance

---

[124] Healthcare Financial Management Association (HFMA), *Price Transparency in Health Care, Report from the HFMA Price Transparency Task Force* (2014), *available at* https://www.hfma.org/transparency/.

[125] *Id.*

[126] U.S. Government Accountability Office (GAO), *Health Care Transparency: Actions Needed to Improve Cost and Quality Information for Consumers*, GAO-15-11, at 11 (Oct. 20, 2014).

[127] Kellogg Insight, *Will People Price Shop for Healthcare?* (Jan. 4, 2018), *available at* https://insight.kellogg.northwestern.edu/article/will-people-price-shop-for-healthcare.

coverage;[128] (2) each patient has unique circumstances that may change the cost of their care;[129] (3) billing for health care services is complex;[130] (4) price information may be more useful to consumers if it also provides them with information about quality;[131] (5) according to one study, less than seven percent of out-of-pocket spending was spent on shoppable health care services;[132] and (6) transparency might be most effective if it is combined with other incentives or benefit designs that encourage consumers to price shop.[133] Section II.B.iv of this memorandum discusses some of these barriers to effective price transparency tools in more detail and highlights some of the recent evidence suggesting that many price transparency initiatives have not been associated with decreased spending.[134]

ii. State Efforts to Promote Transparency of the Cost of Health Care Services for Consumers

As previously mentioned, there are a lot of initiatives at the state level to make the price of health care services available to consumers. For illustrative purposes, below is a non-exhaustive list of some of these efforts.

---

[128] U.S. Government Accountability Office (GAO), *Health Care Transparency: Actions Needed to Improve Cost and Quality Information for Consumers*, GAO-15-11, at 11 (Oct. 20, 2014).

[129] Public Agenda, *Still Searching: How People Use Health Care Price Information in the United States, New York State, Florida, Texas, and New Hampshire* (2017), *available at* https://www.publicagenda.org/files/PublicAgenda_StillSearching_2017.pdf.

[130] Matt Kuhrt, *Report: This is the biggest barrier to consumer price shopping in healthcare*, FIERCEHEALTHCARE (Apr. 11, 2018), *available at* https://www.fiercehealthcare.com/hospitals-health-systems/report-finds-barriers-to- use-price-transparency-tools.

[131] Francois de Brantes, et al., *Price Transparency & Physician Quality Report Card 2017*, ALTARUM AND CATALYST FOR PAYMENT REFORM (2017).

[132] Health Care Cost Institute (HCCI), *Issue Brief: Spending on Shoppable Services in Health Care* (Mar. 2016), *available at* http://www.healthcostinstitute.org/files/Shoppable%20Services%20IB%203.2.16_0.pdf.

[133] *See, e.g., Sunita Desai, et al., Offering A Price Transparency Tool Did Not Reduce Overall Spending Among California Public Employees and Retirees*, HEALTH AFFAIRS 36:8 (Aug. 2017).

[134] Ateev Mehrotra, M.D., M.P.H., Michael E. Chernew, Ph.D, and Anna D. Sinaiko, Ph.D., *Promise and Reality of Price Transparency*, THE NEW ENGLAND JOURNAL OF MEDICINE (Apr. 8, 2018).

- ***New Hampshire***: New Hampshire has adopted robust price transparency policies. New Hampshire created an All-Payer Claims Database (APCD)[135] in 2003 to collect and disseminate information about health care prices.[136] Four years later, in 2007, New Hampshire launched a public website, NHHealthCost.org, that originally provided the median bundled prices for about thirty of the most common health care services.[137] Today, NHHealthCost.org has been expanded to provide consumers with information for over 100 services and provides information about specific providers that can be customized to include information about the individual's specific health plan.[138] The website also includes certain quality information.[139] Additional information about New Hampshire's website and the methodology used for health costs is available on NHHealthCost.org.[140] On July 12, the New Hampshire Insurance Department announced that it was partnering with Harvard Medical School to help New Hampshire residents find medical cost estimates.[141] In the press release, the President and CEO of the Greater Manchester Chamber of Commerce commented that "NHHealthCost.org gives employers a way to share information on the differences in healthcare costs and

[135] Additional information about All-Payer Claims Databases (APCDs) and how they are used to provide consumers with price information is available on a website created by the APCD Council. *See* APCD Council, *APCD Showcase* (last visited Jul. 12, 2018), *available at* https://www.apcdshowcase.org.

[136] The Source on Healthcare Price & Competition, New Hampshire (last visited Jul. 12, 2018), *available at* http://sourceonhealthcare.org/new-hampshire/.

[137] *Id.*

[138] Ateev Mehrotra, M.D., M.P.H., Michael E. Chernew, Ph.D, and Anna D. Sinaiko, Ph.D., *Promise and Reality of Price Transparency*, THE NEW ENGLAND JOURNAL OF MEDICINE (Apr. 8, 2018); New Hampshire Insurance Department, *NH HealthCost* (last visited Jul. 12, 2018), *available at* https://nhhealthcost.nh.gov/costs/medical/step-2/?carrier=uninsured#filter-control.

[139] New Hampshire Insurance Department, *NH HealthCost* (last visited Jul. 12, 2018), *available at* https://nhhealthcost.nh.gov/costs/medical/step-2/?carrier=uninsured#filter-control.

[140] *See* New Hampshire Insurance Department, *Methodology for Health Costs for Consumers* (Jul. 12, 2018), *available at* https://nhhealthcost.nh.gov/methodology-health-costs-consumers.

[141] New Hampshire Insurance Department, *NH Insurance Department Partners with Harvard Medical School to Help NH Residents Find Medical Cost Estimates* (Jul. 12, 2018), *available at* https://www.nh.gov/insurance/media/pr/2018/documents/07-12-18-nh-healthcost-updates-harvard-press-release.pdf.

quality. It also offers resources for large and small employers to help them evaluate the value of their investments in health benefits."[142] New Hampshire also requires that health insurers provide their members with price information.[143]

- ***Massachusetts***: Massachusetts has introduced several bills to improve transparency.[144] One of the price transparency initiatives in Massachusetts was the development of a website that provides consumers with certain information about pricing of different health care services, quality information, and other resources such as suggested questions to ask about health care.[145] The website, MassCompareCare.gov, provides information about the total amount that was paid to the provider for certain services, and allows consumers to compare the costs of medical procedures in different health care facilities.[146] It provides information about the cost of nearly 300 common medical services and procedures.[147] The website also directs consumers to their insurance plan to learn what the procedure will cost them.[148] Under the Massachusetts Healthcare Cost Containment and Quality Improvement law, passed in 2012, all health insurers in Massachusetts are required to provide members with cost estimates online.[149] Recently, Massachusetts announced that it plans to release all of the data it

---

[142] *Id.*

[143] National Conference of State Legislatures, *Transparency and Disclosure of Health Costs and Provider Payments: State Actions* (last updated Mar. 2017), *available at* http://www.ncsl.org/research/health/transparency-and- disclosure-health-costs.aspx.

[144] The Source on Healthcare Price & Competition, *Massachusetts* (last visited Jul. 12, 2018), *available at* http://sourceonhealthcare.org/massachusetts/.

[145] Commonwealth of Massachusetts, *CompareCare* (last visited Jul. 12, 2017), *available at* https://masscomparecare.gov/.

[146] Commonwealth of Massachusetts, *About CompareCare* (last visited Jul. 12, 2017), https://masscomparecare.gov/about.

[147] Priyanka Dayal McCulskey, *What consumers need to know about the state's new health care website*, THE BOSTON GLOBE (May 16, 2018), *available at* https://www.bostonglobe.com/metro/2018/05/15/what-consumers- need-know-about-state-new-health-care-website/n9XGrgu1VtN4mhJQqc8PFL/story.html.

[148] Commonwealth of Massachusetts, *CompareCare* (last visited Jul. 12, 2017), *available at* https://masscomparecare.gov/.

[149] Mass.gov, Mass Consumer Affairs Blog, *Massachusetts Health Insurers Now Required to Provide Prices in Real- Time* (Oct. 1, 2014), *available at* https://blog.mass.gov/consumer/ massconsumer/massachusetts-health-insurers- now-required-to-provide-prices-in-real-time/.

uses to support its website as a single dataset on July 20, 2018, and, at that time, will also launch a transparency data challenge to promote innovative uses of the data.[150]

- ***Ohio***: In 2015, Ohio passed a law requiring providers to give patients a "good faith" estimate of how much non-emergency, elective health care services would cost individuals after accounting for insurance.[151] Due to ongoing litigation, the law has not yet been implemented.[152]
- ***Colorado***: Colorado has passed many proposals to promote price transparency.[153] One of the recent initiatives passed by Colorado requires that hospitals and certain other provider groups to post their private-pay, non-discounted fees on their websites, or make them available upon request, for the most common health care services that they provide.[154]
- ***Illinois***: Illinois has implemented several policies to promote price transparency.[155] One of the laws passed in Illinois requires that hospitals give prospective patients estimated costs of services before treatment.[156]

Again, the above list is just a sampling of some of the state initiatives. For example, other states with health care price transparency websites

---

[150] Center for Health Information and Analysis (CHIA), Strategy for Releasing Procedure Price Data (Jun. 2018), available at http://www.chiamass.gov/assets/Uploads/Strategy-for-Releasing-Procedure-Pricing-Data.pdf.

[151] The Source on Healthcare Price & Competition, *Ohio* (last visited Jul. 12, 2018), *available at* http://sourceonhealthcare.org/ohio/.

[152] *Id.*

[153] The Source on Healthcare Price & Competition, *Colorado* (last visited Jul. 12, 2018), *available at* http://sourceonhealthcare.org/legislation-regulation/colorado/.

[154] Colorado General Assembly, *SB17-065: Transparency in Direct Pay Health Care Prices* (2017), *available at* https://leg.colorado.gov/bills/sb17-065; *See also* Richard Mark Kirkner, *If You Make Them Build It, They Still May Not Come*, MANAGED CARE (Jun. 3, 2018), *available at* https://www.managedcaremag.com/archives/2018/6/if-you- make-them-build-it-they-still-may-not-come.

[155] The Source on Healthcare Price & Competition, *Illinois* (last visited Jul. 12, 2018), *available at* http://sourceonhealthcare.org/illinois/.

[156] National Conference of State Legislatures, Tr*ansparency and Disclosure of Health Costs and Provider Statements: State Actions* (last updated Mar. 2017), *available at* http://www.ncsl.org/research/health/transparency- and-disclosure-health-costs.aspx.

include, but are not limited to, Oregon,[157] Maine,[158] Maryland,[159] and Washington.[160] While there have been several state initiatives targeted at price transparency, an annual report card released by the Catalyst for Payment Reform and Altarum's Center for Payment Innovation still gives most states a failing grade.[161] Indeed, in the 2017 report card, only two states—Maine and New Hampshire—received an "A" for transparency, only two states—Maryland and Oregon—received a "B" for transparency, and only three states—Colorado, Vermont, and Virginia—received a "C" for transparency. The other 43 states received an "F" for transparency.[162] According to the organizations, "states with high price transparency grades have rich data sources and supply meaningful price information on a wide range of procedures and services that is presented on an accessible, publicly available website."[163]

States have encountered a lot of different barriers while trying to adopt some of these transparency initiatives. For example, many of the state transparency websites utilize information from the state's All-Payer Claims Databases (APCDs) to help facilitate price shopping, and there have been a number of implementation challenges for APCDs including issues relating to: (1) concerns with data privacy and security; (2) concerns with the accuracy and integrity of the data that is submitted and whether the data conveys information in an accurate manner; (3) concerns with the comprehensiveness of the data submitted to the APCD; (4) concerns regarding whether the release of negotiated price information could violate

---

[157] OregonHospitalGuide.org (last visited Jul. 12, 2018), *available at* http://oregonhospital guide.org/.

[158] CompareMaine.org (last visited Jul. 12, 2018), *available at* http://www.comparemaine.org.

[159] Maryland Health Care Commission, *Wear the Cost* (last visited Jul. 12, 2018), *available at* http://wearthecost.org; *See also* Robert E. Moffitt, Ph.D, et al., *The Next Chapter In Transparency: Maryland's Wear the Cost*, THE HERITAGE FOUNDATION (Oct. 19, 2017), *available at* https://www.heritage.org/health-care-reform/commentary/the- next-chapter-transparency-marylands-wear-the-cost.

[160] Washington HealthCareCompare (last visited Jul. 12, 2018), *available at* https://www.wahealthcarecompare.com.

[161] In 2017, the Catalyst for Payment Reform and Altarum's Center for Payment Innovation issued a report card that combined price transparency and quality information in one report card. Francois de Brantes, et al., *Price Transparency & Physician Quality Report Card 2017*, ALTARUM AND CATALYST FOR PAYMENT REFORM (2017).

[162] *Id.*

[163] *Id.* at 3.

state and federal antitrust laws and lead to collusion; (5) concerns that the requested information is confidential information pursuant to specific contractual provisions or is subject to trade secret protection; and (6) concerns with the administrative cost to comply with some of the requirements.[164]

iii. Other Price Transparency Tools that are Available to Promote Transparency of Health Care Services for Consumers

The private sector has also pursued a lot of different transparency efforts to help inform consumers of the price of health care services. Nearly all insurers provide their members with access to a health care cost transparency tool.[165] Many employers—at least 85 percent of self-insured employers according to one report—also use vendors such as Castlight Health and Truven Health Analytics to provide health care price transparency tools to employees.[166] According to a poll conducted by one of these vendors, Truven, 80 percent of the individuals who used the tool and were surveyed said that the cost transparency tool "helped them understand their financial responsibility up front."[167] Similarly, some hospitals and other providers have developed health care price transparency tools for patients.[168]

---

[164] The Source on Healthcare Price & Competition, *Healthcare Legislative Topics: All Payer Claims Databases*, MEDIUM (Apr. 3, 2015), *available at* https://medium.com/@SourceOnHealth/healthcare-legislative-topics-all-payer- claims-databases-6f87b24c7fcf.

[165] Shelby Livingston, *Is the price right? Solving healthcare's transparency problem*, MODERN HEALTHCARE (last visited Jul. 12, 2018), *available at* http://www.modernhealthcare.com/reports/achieving-transparency-in-healthcare/#!/.

[166] *Id.*

[167] Truven Health Analytics, *The Value of Price Transparency in Healthcare* (last visited Jul. 14, 2018), *available at* http://img.en25.com/Web/TruvenHealthAnalytics/Price_Transparency_Infographic_FINAL.pdf.

[168] *See, e.g.*, Harris Meyer, Hospitals roll out online price estimators as CMS presses for transparency, Modern Healthcare (Jun. 23, 2018), available at http://www.modernhealthcare.com/article/20180623/NEWS/180629994.

C. Role and Impact of Health Care Price Transparency

As previously mentioned, there has been an increasing amount of interest in the role of price transparency, especially as consumers are directly responsible for more of their health care costs.[169] Patients generally want to know how much health care services will cost. A report released by Public Agenda in 2017 found that about 50 percent of Americans have tried to find health care price information before obtaining care and about 20 percent of individuals have tried to compare provider prices.[170] A report released by the Foundation for Government Accountability (FGA) found that 77 percent of Americans want the "Right to Shop" in health care.[171] Having access to price and quality information can help enable patients identify lower cost and high quality care.[172]

While these reports showed that many patients want to know the cost of their health care services, some other studies have raised concerns about how, if at all, consumers use some of the available price transparency tools.[173] In April 2018, the *New England Journal of Medicine* published an article entitled "Promise and Reality of Price Transparency" that described how "[m]any politicians and experts believe that price transparency will increase price shopping and reduce health care spending," yet concluded that "[t]o date, price transparency has not achieved the promises of facilitating price shopping and decreasing spending."[174] The article reasoned that price transparency tools may not have encouraged price

---

[169] *See, e.g.*, U.S. Government Accountability Office (GAO), *Health Care Transparency: Actions Needed to Improve Cost and Quality Information for Consumers*, GAO-15-11, at 1 (Oct. 20, 2014).

[170] Public Agenda, *Still Searching: How People Use Health Care Price Information in the United States, New York State, Florida, Texas, and New Hampshire* (Apr. 2017).

[171] Foundation for Government Accountability, *Allies of Right to Shop: Paying Patients to Pick High-Value Healthcare* (Dec. 28, 2016), *available at* https://thefga.org/research/allies-of-right-to-shop-2/.

[172] *See, e.g.*, Foundation for Government Accountability, *How a Patient Experiences Right to Shop – Jenny's Story* (Dec. 28, 2016), *available at* https://thefga.org/research/how-a-patient-experiences-right-to-shop-2/.

[173] Ateev Mehrotra, MD, MPH, et al., *Defining Goals of Health Care Price Transparency: Not Just Shopping Around*, NEJM CATALYST (Jun. 26, 2018), *available at* https://catalyst.nejm.org/health-care-price-transparency- goals/.

[174] Ateev Mehrotra, M.D., M.P.H., Michael E. Chernew, Ph.D, and Anna D. Sinaiko, Ph.D., *Promise and Reality of Price Transparency*, THE NEW ENGLAND JOURNAL OF MEDICINE (Apr. 8, 2018).

shopping because many patients do not know about the available tools, the complexity of health care billing makes it difficult for patients to price shop, patients are not given standardized information that they can use to make price comparisons, most health plans do not have benefit designs that encourage price shopping, and patients do not want to disrupt their relationship with their provider.[175] Another article highlighted that there are many different purposes for price transparency, and determining the success of different price transparency efforts depends on the goal trying to be accomplished.[176] Similarly, some experts have questioned whether consumers are the best target of transparency efforts or, alternatively, if transparency targeted at other stakeholders, such as providers, would be more effective.[177]

In addition to concerns about whether consumers are using price transparency tools and whether they decrease spending, some experts have cautioned that it is important to carefully structure price transparency initiatives to avoid unintentional consequences. For example, during a 2014 workshop at the Federal Trade Commission (FTC) examining health care competition and efforts to provide consumers, providers, payers, employers, and other stakeholders with meaningful price transparency, some of the panelists discussed how some forms of price transparency might have unintended consequences such as leading consumers to more expensive providers.[178] Similarly, in a July 2015 blog post, the FTC cautioned that "transparency is not universally good," and if it "goes too far, it can actually harm competition and consumers."[179]

---

[175] *Id.*

[176] Ateev Mehrotra, MD, MPH, et al., *Defining Goals of Health Care Price Transparency: Not Just Shopping Around*, NEJM CATALYST (Jun. 26, 2018), *available at* https://catalyst.nejm.org/health-care-price-transparency- goals/.

[177] *See, e.g., id.*

[178] Federal Trade Commission, *Workshop Transcript: Examining Health Care Competition*, at 85-6 (Mar. 21, 2014), *available at* https://www.ftc.gov/system/files/documents/public_events/200361/transcriptmar21_0.pdf.

[179] Tara Isa Koslov and Elizabeth Jex, Office of Policy Planning, Federal Trade Commission, *Price transparency or TMI?* (Jul. 2, 2015), *available at* https://www.ftc.gov/news-events/blogs/competition-matters/2015/07/price- transparency-or-tmi.

iii. Issues

The following issues may be examined at the hearing:

- Different state efforts to enhance price transparency and provide consumers with information about the cost of medical care and medical products;
- The purposes of different price transparency tools that states have adopted to provide consumers with information about the cost of medical care;
- How to most effectively provide consumers with meaningful price information that they can use to evaluate medical care;
- Concerns with some of the different price transparency efforts that have been pursued at the state level;
- Whether consumers have been using some of the various price transparency tools, and if not, the reasons that consumers have not been using them; and
- Whether there are other forms of transparency, such as transparency directed at providers rather than consumers, that should also be considered.

iv. Staff Contacts

If you have any questions regarding the hearing, please contact Jen Barblan, Natalie Turner, or Lamar Echols of the Committee staff at (202) 225-2927.

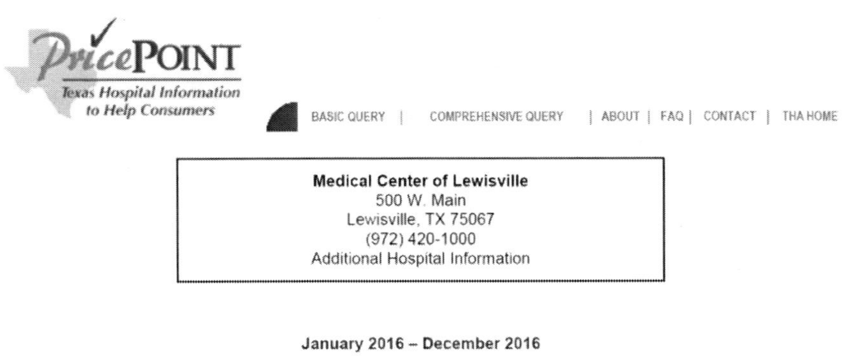

	Selected Hospital	All Hospitals in this County	Hospitals with Similar Patient Care	All Texas Hospitals
Number of Discharges:	287	843	72,046	84,939
Average Length-of-Stay:	3.5 Day(s)	3.1 Day(s)	2.8 Day(s)	2.8 Day(s)
Average Charge:	$28,364	$22,800	$24,131	$23,786
Average Charge Per Day:	$8,104	$7,355	$8,618	$8,495
Median Charge:	$26,201	$21,935	$21,892	$21,836

NR = 1 - 4 Discharges (Not Reported)
= Show hospitals in that group

- Notes About this Table
- Understanding Hospital Charge Information
- Why Charges May Differ Between Hospitals

[Select New Hospital] [Select New Service at this Hospital]

MEDICAL CENTER OF LEWISVILLE
CHARGE AND PAYMENT INFORMATION
MOST RECENT FISCAL YEAR - ALL SERVICES

What is the selected hospital's "payer mix?"
A hospital's "payer mix" refers to the proportion of its total charges attributable to different types of insurance coverage.

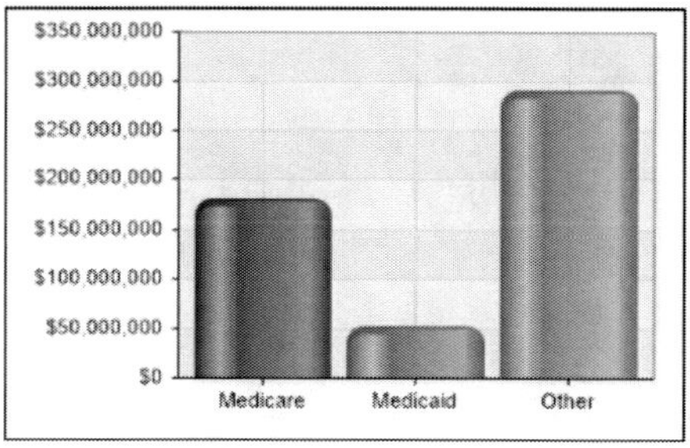

Medicare
Medicaid
Other

How much do government programs pay compared to private insurance?
In many cases, Medicare & Medicaid reimburse hospitals at rates that do not cover the costs they incur to provide care. Payments from privately insured patients generally subsidize the shortfalls created by Medicare and Medicaid and therefore represent a "hidden tax" on individuals and families not covered by government programs.

The graphs below represent all services provided by the hospital; they are not specific to the the selected service.

ALL PAYERS*
This hospital collects an average of **27%** of its charges from all payers.

☐ $381,172,861 Charges Not Paid
■ $142,853,482 Charges Paid

MEDICARE*
This hospital collects an average of **16%** of its charges from Medicare.

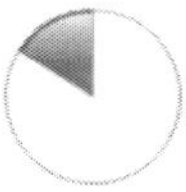

☐ $151,719,915 Charges Not Paid
■ $29,158,372 Charges Paid

**Payments determined by federal government*

MEDICAID*
This hospital collects an average of **17%** of its charges from Medicaid.

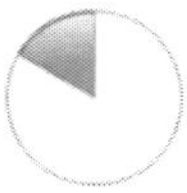

☐ $43,178,707 Charges Not Paid
■ $8,693,669 Charges Paid

**excludes Medicaid Disproportionate Share and UPL payments*

The above information is for <u>all services</u> at the selected hospital. It is not specific to the service you selected or any other single service. Contact your insurer to determine the specific amount that will be paid under your policy for the selected service.

The table below details the health care charges that the hospital did not receive payment for because the patient qualified for free or reduced-charge care or because the patient failed to pay what was owed.

	Charges	Percent of Total Charges
Charity Care:	$5,124,449	0.98%
Bad Debt:	$23,950,252	4.57%
Total Uncompensated Care:	$29,074,701	5.55%

HEALTH AFFAIRS BLOG BUILDING SOMETHING WORTH BUILDING FOR ALL PATIENTS

Michael Burgess

MARCH 24, 2008 DOI: 10.1377/hblog20080324.000367

Editor's Note: *Today, Rep. Michael Burgess (R-TX) kicks off a series of posts on Jon Gabel's article "Where Do I Send Thee? Does Physician-Ownership Affect Referral Patterns To Ambulatory Surgical Centers?," published March 18 on the* Health Affairs *Web site. The series will also feature posts from Jerry Cromwell and Chris Cassel.*

To paraphrase the great American architect, Frank Lloyd Wright: no man should write about building who has not himself built something worth building. As a physician who helped build an ambulatory surgery center (ASC), I conform to Mr. Wright's formula and am glad to pen some thoughts about my personal experiences with the facility.

Let me begin by stipulating that I am neither a statistician, an economist, nor an academic. I have, however, practiced twenty-five years' worth of medicine. My experience is far-ranging: from a multispecialty practice, to a solo practice, and then in a single-specialty group. It was as a part of this single-specialty group I helped organize and start an ASC in my Texas hometown. And now, by virtue of the fact that I have been elected to Congress, one could argue that I've become an expert in almost anything.

Therefore, I am grateful to have the opportunity to provide some alternative insights into the conclusions outlined in the piece by Jon Gabel and colleagues titled "Where Do I Send Thee? Does Physician-Ownership Affect Referral Patterns to Ambulatory Surgery Centers?"

While the overall piece is thoughtful, I take issue with some of the conclusions. First and foremost, it is unfair to assume that self-pay patients fall into one of two categories: those seeking cosmetic surgery or those who are wealthy. There are also those who lack health insurance.

Like other patients, the uninsured require and request surgery as well. In my own practice of obstetrics and gynecology, it was in dealing with patients who lacked health insurance where the payment disparity among different facilities became most apparent. Many times I encountered patients who desired operations, such as tubal ligation, but lacked health insurance. If they chose to pay for this operation, our local hospital would ask them to pay up front between $8,000 and $12,000. If, however, they were to make the same inquiry at an outpatient surgical center, they would find the total facility fee to be in the range of $1,000. My own modest fee for this procedure was in the neighborhood of $400, which would be unchanged whether the surgery was performed in a hospital facility or an ASC.

In response to these facts, I would simply ask the rhetorical question: in which scenario was I more likely to be paid my fee? That in which the patient had paid $1,000 for the facility or a figure about ten times as high? Invariably the patient's finances would be depleted by the hospital charge, and the physician's fee would often go unpaid.

Thus, if a patient with no insurance presented to my practice for an elective procedure, my likelihood of receiving compensation might, in fact, be increased if the patient were referred to an ASC, regardless of ownership.

Ownership Encourages Quality

Payment disparities are certainly a challenge. But, there are many other health care concerns today, including the issues of quality of care and payment for performance. One of the most controversial and complex subjects is physician-ownership of medical facilities, as evidenced by Gabel and colleagues' discussion. There is an old axiom that says no one ever checks the water in the battery of a rental car. There is a lot to be said for pride of ownership in any facility, including one's own office or one's ASC.

The Relative Efficiency of ASCs

Paperwork and policy are also problems when it comes to modern-day health care. In my own twenty-five years of clinical practice, I had multiple struggles with hospital administration. Indeed, sometimes the conventional wisdom was that my local hospital behaved like an absentee landlord. I recall very vividly a five-year effort to get filtered drinking water for my hospitalized patients. It is not a battle I would like to relive at any point in the future.

Additionally, timing and schedules are critical parts of any medical practice. I was fortunate to have a robust roster of patients. So I began scheduling minor procedures on a day that I typically took out of the office. If I were to do four procedures at my local hospital, turnover time after each case would approach one hour. As a consequence, I could complete those four extra cases each week, but it would consume a large amount of time.

If, however, those four cases were performed in an ASC, turnover time was much shorter. It allowed me to place the patient safely in the recovery room, speak with her family, and dictate a procedure note before it was time to start the next case. This meant that those four cases could be accomplished by mid-morning and I could be off about other pursuits.

Turnover time was reduced because the correct incentives were in place to make the facility run smoothly and safely.

The Need for Better Data on Physician Owners of ASCs

While I disagree with several of Gabel and colleagues' assertions, I do concur with their statements about the difficulty in interpretation of data because of the lack of public information about physician owners of ambulatory surgery centers. In fact, without this relevant data, any conclusion drawn becomes suspect – relying on broad generalities, or merely reinforcing preconceived notions. It is frequently hard to correct for observer bias.

Additionally, the statements on the difference between Medicaid and Blue Cross Blue Shield – in other words, those ranging from the lowest to the highest payer – were somewhat confusing. As a clinician, why would I want to invest more of my most valuable commodity (time) to treat a patient for which my reimbursement is lowest? In the interest of precious time, it seems that the incentive for treating the Medicaid patient would be tilted toward the ASCs, so that it could be done more efficiently. Whenever I am confronted with a set of medical choices, my first default question is always, "Is it safe?" Secondly, I might consider, "What is the least complicated option for me and my patient?" And third, "What are the clinical as well as the business outcomes?" Thus, if I found myself recommending a procedure for a patient, and it could be safely performed in a surgery center, regardless of the amount of available compensation, the ease of scheduling and the rapidity of performance would tend to influence me toward the outpatient facility.

There also might be a case to be made in terms of differentiation by specialties. Generalists such as gynecologists or general surgeons will typically have a broad mix of patients.

Their diagnoses might reveal a different pattern than those among physicians who were more narrowly focused within a more well-defined specialty.

Differing Attitudes toward the Provision of Health Care

Finally, within the discussion section for this piece, perhaps the focus should not be on why the lowest reimbursement patients (Medicaid) were referred least often to an ASC. Instead, we should determine why Medicaid is the lowest payer. We should also explore what this says about those who want to expand the government's role in paying for health care.

The paper talks about 11 a.m. on a Sunday morning. The statement is made that this might be the most segregated hour of the week. I am not certain about the source of that data, but I do wonder if there is a mindset of a segment of the population who believe that they should pay nothing for medical care versus those who search for an affordable option when hospital costs have increased to a level would preclude their use.

The fact remains that both hospitals and ASCs are necessary for providing good, efficient, and cost-effective care in modern medicine. Physicians are more inherently aware of this fact than any other profession. Therefore, it is not surprising that they would want to provide these types of facilities or partner with their hospitals to provide these types of facilities, to provide the best possible care for their patients in an efficient and cost-effective manner. After all, it is patient care that really matters at the end of the day, and this begins and ends with doctors.

NCPA - National Community Pharmacists Association

July 17, 2018

The Honorable Buddy Carter

United States House of Representatives

432 Cannon House Office Building

Washington, DC 20515

Dear Representative Carter:

The National Community Pharmacists Association wishes to thank the House Energy and Commerce Committee's Subcommittee on Oversight and Investigations for conducting this hearing, "Examining State Efforts to Improve Transparency of Health Care Costs for Consumers." This is a vital hearing looking at health care price transparency that has emerged as a hot topic in state government and legislatures as a strategy for containing health costs for consumers and state governments. NCPA would like to share our experiences with states that have enacted legislation and initiated programs that aim to reduce costs and bring about increased transparency to the drug pricing system.

NCPA represents America's community pharmacists, including the owners of more than 22,000 independent community pharmacies. Together they represent an $80 billion health care marketplace and employ more than 250,000 individuals on a full or part-time basis. Independent community pharmacies are also typically located in traditionally underserved rural and urban communities, providing critical access to residents of these communities.

Community pharmacists have long been concerned with pharmacy benefit managers (PBMs) operating as largely unregulated middlemen in the drug supply chain. While PBMs claim to keep drug costs low, we believe PBM practices are anti-competitive and ultimately drive up healthcare costs for consumers and plan sponsors while reducing payments to pharmacies.

PBMs determine which pharmacies patients may choose by creating provider networks, determine which drugs patients can be prescribed by creating drug formularies, and determine how much patients pay at the pharmacy counter for their medications. Despite their authority over patients' health care options, PBMs enjoy little regulatory oversight by the state.

State Efforts to Increase PBM Transparency in the Medicaid Program

Spurred by patient concerns, policymakers in several states have examined PBM practices and contract management in their Medicaid managed care programs. Those policymakers have found Medicaid managed care organizations (MCOs) that fail to hold their PBMs accountable, narrow networks that limit patient access to trusted community pharmacists, PBMs that often pay themselves much more than they pay community pharmacies, and spread pricing models that disadvantage taxpayers. Having examined the role of PBMs, policymakers in some states are implementing reforms in their Medicaid managed care programs to correct these abuses.

For example, in the summer of 2017, West Virginia carved pharmacy benefits out of its Medicaid managed care program. The state's Department of Health and Human Resources made the move after an actuarial study showed that Medicaid could save $30 million annually by administering the benefit directly, and that doing so would also put $34 million back into local economies in the form of pharmacy reimbursements. Anecdotal reports from Medicaid officials indicate that the actual savings thus far are in line with the projections.

In Kentucky, the state spends approximately $1.68 billion of taxpayer funds on the pharmacy benefit in the Medicaid managed care program. While testifying in front of legislative committees, the state Medicaid administrator could not explain where that money was going, other than it was going to MCOs. Data shows that as much as $380 million could be going directly into the pockets of the PBMs. This lack of transparency and accountability drew the ire of legislators who soon thereafter enacted some of the strongest Medicaid transparency language in the country. Under the new law, Kentucky's Department for Medicaid Services has the authority to review and approve contracts between an MCO and its PBM, contracts between a PBM administering Medicaid drug benefits and a pharmacy, and PBM reimbursement rates.

The law also requires PBMs to disclose the difference between the amount the pharmacy is reimbursed for filling a prescription and the amount the PBM charges the MCO for administering the claim.

Kentucky is not the only state to take action and increase transparency by examining PBMs' spread pricing models. Virginia and Georgia have also passed legislation requiring PBMs to disclose the difference between the amount the pharmacy is reimbursed for filling a prescription and the amount the PBM charges the MCO for administering the claim. Similarly, in Ohio and Pennsylvania, the state auditors have announced plans to review PBM practices in those states' Medicaid managed care programs and investigate potential wrongdoing after realizing that community pharmacies' reimbursements have been decreasing, but overall state spending on prescription drugs continues to increase.

Conclusion

Members of this subcommittee should be just as concerned as state policymakers have been in realizing how harmful a lack of transparency is when it comes to PBMs' use of public tax dollars. MCOs have not been holding PBMs accountable, and states are beginning to take control. Those states have learned that constant vigilance and increased transparency is necessary to keep PBMs honest and ensure public funds are spent properly. These measures not only protect taxpayers' wallets, but they ensure that Medicaid beneficiaries can continue accessing the services of trusted community pharmacists. The success of these and similar initiatives have been noticed by states and organizations across the country, including the National Council of Insurance Legislators, which is currently developing model PBM transparency legislation. While examining efforts to improve transparency of health care costs of consumers, the committee should pay close attention to the success that states have had by increasing PBM transparency.

Sincerely,

Karry K. La Violette
Senior Vice President
Government Affairs and Director of Advocacy Center

In: Health Care Costs for Consumers … ISBN: 978-1-53616-862-4
Editor: Maik Nacht

Chapter 2

SMALL BUSINESS HEALTH CARE: COSTS AND OPTIONS*

Subcommittee on Primary Health and Retirement Security

Tuesday, June 28, 2016

U.S. Senate, Subcommittee on Primary Health and Retirement Security, Committee on Health, Education, Labor, and Pensions, Washington, DC.

The subcommittee met, pursuant to notice, at 2:05 p.m., in room SD–430, Dirksen Senate Office Building, Hon. Michael Enzi, chairman of the subcommittee, presiding.

Present: Senators Enzi, Scott, Cassidy, Murphy, and Bennet.

---

* This is an edited, reformatted and augmented version of Hearing Before the Subcommittee on Primary Health and Retirement Security of the Committee on Health, Education, Labor, and Pensions United States Senate, One Hundred Fourteenth Congress, Second Session, Publication No. S. HRG. 114–782, dated 2018.

OPENING STATEMENT OF SENATOR ENZI

Senator ENZI. I'll go ahead and call to order this HELP Subcommittee on Primary Health and Retirement Security roundtable, at a square table, but this is as close as we come to round around here. I got word from Senator Sanders to go ahead.

I'll do my opening statement, and when he gets here, he can do his opening statement, and if he isn't here by the time I finish, then we'll go ahead and start having you give a summary of your testimony, and then following that, we'll have the discussion and questions.

I'd like to thank all of you for coming today, and I'd like to thank the staffs on both sides of the aisle for working on putting together a bipartisan conversation about what's important to small business in the area of healthcare. I'd also like to thank all my colleagues for being interested in this and ready to engage in important discussion. There will be more here throughout the afternoon.

I think we have here at the table representation from many experts who have a valuable perspective about what the reality is for small businesses helping their employees purchase health insurance. I'm anxius to get to the real discussion, but I'd like to touch on the heart of what I hope we can get to today.

Small businesses are the backbone of our economy. In Wyoming today, we're watching our communities being decimated by the collapse of the energy sector. Thousands of jobs have been lost, but, as you know, those losses never happen in isolation. Main street businesses feel the hit with their customers. They feel the crunch of a down economy, and we have to consider what additional pressures they have to face.

Small businesses as a whole are different than big businesses. Despite the fact that they're not legally required to offer health insurance, so many small employers do. Offering health insurance helps give their business a competitive advantage and incentivizes employee retention, but many employers also offer health insurance plans out of a sense of responsibility to their employees.

We want employers to stay involved in the health of their employees. But Washington has done nearly everything possible to make it a bad business decision to continue to offer health insurance options. Policymakers often want to be supportive of small businesses but may not truly understand the challenges they actually have on the ground.

I know that when I was running my small shoe store, I found out that any business that I looked at looked easy to operate, so long as I didn't have to get behind the counter and run it. People don't realize the decisions that have to be made, how long in advance they have to be made, how you train people, how you acquire people, and how difficult all that is. You may be the owner of a small business, but you're also usually the same person who opens the store, who waits on the customers, who cleans the bathroom, who stocks the merchandise, all while trying to meet payroll every week and keep up on any new government regulations.

I also know the amazing satisfaction you get when you see your business take off, the point where you think that you're really going to make it work. The business owners I know see that as a shared success with their employees. It's a community. You know their families. You want to make sure those people are taken care of.

The Federal Government has tried a variety of approaches to fix the small group market. There's general agreement that we still aren't there yet, and some would say that we've made things worse. Today, I'd like to focus the discussion on the biggest challenge for small businesses wishing to help their employees with health care, and that cost. It's the No. 1 reason that small businesses say they do not provide health insurance assistance for their employees. This is not a discussion about one particular bill or priority. I'd ask our panel today to think beyond what the market was before the Affordable Care Act and what it is under the Affordable Care Act. We need to look at what small businesses actually want in the next 10 to 15 years. That translates into affordable options with more flexibility and fewer restrictions.

The landscape in healthcare has rapidly changed. We must be willing to consider a variety of options. Perhaps it should not resemble today's market at all. If we try to fit health insurance into an outdated mold with priorities and sacred cows of a decade ago, we won't be able to make much progress.

I think we agree here that cost is a problem. If the Federal Gov ernment has created an affordability problem or exacerbated it, we should identify it and figure out how to fix it. Our government is even more deeply embedded in healthcare now than ever, and we're seeing the impact of that in rising premiums and tighter family budgets.

Just to clarify the process, after Senator Sanders speaks or prior to him being here, I'll ask each of the participants to speak briefly. You've submitted statements. Your entire statement will be a matter of record for this roundtable. After your introductory comments, if you'd like to respond to something that's been said or one of the questions that we ask, if you'd just stand your name tag up on end, we'll know to call on you and we'll try to keep track of the order of that.

First, I'd like to welcome a fellow Wyomingite, Tom Glause, who is the Insurance Commissioner in Wyoming. He has firsthand knowledge of the insurance markets and how policies impact costs. I also understand that you have an accounting degree. I'm always glad to see that. There are two of us in the Senate.

Next is Warren Hudak. Mr. Hudak is the president of Hudak and Company, an accounting firm in Cumberland, PA. He has seven employees and has personal experience in purchasing health insurance as a small employer.

I appreciate you taking time away from your business to participate.

I want to welcome Mr. Thomas Harte. He's the president of Landmark Benefits in New Hampshire. Mr. Harte's company provides employee benefit services to over 300 corporations and thousands of employees.

You have participated in our roundtable before, and I appreciate you coming back again.

Ms. Sarah Lueck is Senior Policy Analyst at the Center on Budget Policy and Priorities here in Washington, DC. Ms. Lueck works on issues related to health reform implementation, specifically, health insurance exchanges and private market reforms included. I want to thank you all for your time. Also, another thing that we do is at the conclusion, we allow a short period of time for people to submit written questions that we would hope that you'd be willing to answer as well, and those become a part of the record, too.

At this point in time, we'll go ahead and begin the discussion, and if each of you would summarize your comments, which will be in the record completely, we'd appreciate it. That leaves more time for more questions and comments.

We'll begin with you, Mr. Glause.

STATEMENT OF TOM GLAUSE, COMMISSIONER, WYOMING DEPARTMENT OF INSURANCE, CHEYENNE, WY

Mr. GLAUSE. Good afternoon, Chairman Enzi and members of the Subcommittee on Primary Health and Retirement Security. Thank you for asking me to participate in this Roundtable Discussion on Small Business Health Care: Costs and Options. My name is Tom Glause. I am the Insurance Commissioner for the State of Wyoming.

As the least populated State in our Nation, Wyoming faces challenges in providing health insurance coverage for its citizens. Since the passage of the ACA, a large number of health insurance companies have left the Wyoming market. Currently, Wyoming has only one insurer participating in the Federal marketplace for both individuals and small group plans.

The exodus from the health insurance market has been for a variety of reasons, including financial insolvency, changing focus of product lines, and effects of the ACA. As the State is currently experiencing an economic downturn, employers are reporting that they must reduce or cut employer provided health insurance in order to maintain employment positions.

We have seen a slow but steady increase in the number of par ticipants in the individual marketplace, but very little participation in the SHOP plans. As of May 31st, Wyoming's only SHOP carrier reports just 103 contracts covering less than 300 lives. Wyoming has traditionally had the highest rate of employerprovided healthcare coverage in the Nation. According to the Kaiser Family Foundation, in 2014, the national average for employer-sponsored health plans was 49 percent, whereas Wyoming was 61 percent.

The mandated coverage for essential health benefits has been costly and burdensome on small employers. Wyoming employers report that they want to provide coverage for their employees but feel constrained by the cost and the requirements that the small group plans must contain the ACA's 10 essential health benefits.

In 2015, the Wyoming State legislature passed statutory language to clarify that if a small employer offers coverage to its employees, the employer has the option of offering coverage to the employees' dependents. In some cases, this legislative change has allowed the employees' dependents to obtain individual coverage on the marketplace.

Network adequacy continues to be an issue. It was before the ACA, and it remains an issue today. Wyoming only has 196.7 physicians per 100,000 residents, compared to an average of 265.5 nationally. In addition, Wyoming covers almost 98,000 square miles. Needless to say, our providers are widely scattered.

Uncompensated care remains a concern in nearly all care facilities in our State. A May 2016 report from the Wyoming Hospital Association indicates a 3 percent annual increase in uncompensated care. The Association anticipates larger increases because of increasing unemployment, an increasing number of high deductible health insurance plans, and an increasing number of uninsureds. Wyoming has the second highest premium rates in the Nation, second only to Alaska. On the individual market, in 2016, the average monthly premium before the advanced premium tax credit was $571, compared to the national average of $396. Wyoming employers have reported that the tax benefits of providing coverage are often difficult and convoluted. Others report that it's less expensive to pay the tax than to provide health insurance coverage.

The Wyoming Small Employer Reinsurance Plan has begun a runout of the program and the claims. The number of ceded lives into the plan has continued to decline, indicating a decreasing number of small employer sponsored plans.

In conclusion, there are two primary considerations for small businesses when considering whether to provide health insurance to its employees. The first is cost: the cost of the premiums to the employer and the employee and the cost of time in administering the program. The second is choice. Can the small employers provide coverage that their employees need with networks that are sufficient and out-of-pocket costs that are reasonable?

Thank you for inviting me to this roundtable discussion, and I look forward to your questions.

[The prepared statement of Mr. Glause follows:]

Prepared Statement of Tom Glause

Good afternoon, Chairman Enzi and members of the subcommittee on Primary Health and Retirement Security. Thank you for asking me to participate in this Roundtable Discussion on Small Business Health Care: Costs and Options. My name is Tom Glause. I am the Insurance Commissioner for the State of Wyoming, appointed to this position by Governor Matt Mead in January 2015.

As the least populated State in our Nation, Wyoming faces challenges in providing health insurance coverage for its citizens. Perhaps some observations and information about my State may be helpful in discussions regarding small employer plans in general but specifically regarding the small employer market in rural settings. Since the passage of the ACA, a large number of health insurance companies left the Wyoming market. Currently, Wyoming has only one insurer participating in the Federal Marketplace for both individuals and the small group or SHOP plans. The exodus from the health insurance market has been for a variety of reasons, including insurer financial insolvency, changing focus of product lines, and effects of the ACA.

As the State is currently experiencing an economic downturn, employers are selfreporting they must reduce or cut employer provided health insurance in order to maintain employment positions. We have seen a slow but steady increase in the number of participants on the Individual Marketplace but very little participation in the SHOP plans. As of May 31, Wyoming's only SHOP carrier reports just 103 contracts, covering less than 300 lives. The individual Marketplace reports 23,770 enrollees for 2016.

Wyoming has traditionally had the highest rate of employer provided health coverage in the Nation. According to the Kaiser Family Foundation, in 2014, the national average for employer sponsored health plans was 49 percent, whereas Wyoming was 61 percent, followed closely by Maryland at 60 percent.

The mandated coverage of the Essential Health Benefits (EHB) has been costly and burdensome on small employers. Wyoming employers report they want to provide coverage for their employees but feel constrained by cost and the requirement that these small group plans must contain the ACA's 10 Essential Health Benefits. Employers have expressed concern over their desire to provide benefits to their employees and the coverage mandate that is not required of large group employers. In 2015, the Wyoming State Legislature passed statutory language to clarify that if a small employer offers coverage to its employees, the employer has the option of offering coverage to the employee's dependents. Wyo. Stat. § 26–19–306(c)(vi). In some cases, this legislative change allowed the employee's dependents to opt for individual coverage on the Marketplace.

Network Adequacy was an issue before the ACA and remains an issue today. Wyoming reports 196.7 physicians per 100,000 people whereas the national average is 265.5 per 100,000. In addition, Wyoming covers 97,818 square miles—needless to say, our providers are widely scattered.

Uncompensated Care remains a concern in nearly all care facilities in our State. A May 2016 report from the Wyoming Hospital Association indicates at least a 3 percent annual increase in uncompensated care but the association anticipates larger increases because of increasing unemployment, increasing numbers of individuals with high deductible plans, and increasing numbers of uninsured.

Wyoming is a nonrate setting State; therefore, we rely upon the qualified health plan (QHP) determinations and rate approvals conducted by the Center for Medicare and Medicaid Services (CMS). Wyoming has the second highest premium rates in the Nation, second only to Alaska. On the individual market in 2016, the average monthly premium before the Advanced Premium Tax Credit (APTC) was $571 compared to the national average of $396. Some Wyoming employers have reported that the tax benefits for providing coverage are difficult and convoluted. Others report it is less expensive to pay the tax penalties than to provide health insurance coverage.

The Wyoming Small Employer Health Reinsurance Plan (WySEHRP) plan has begun a runout of the program and claims, after it was determined that the number of ceded lives has continued to decline as transitional plans will be exiting the market. The declining number indicate a decreasing number of small employer sponsored plans.

In conclusion, in my opinion, there are two primary considerations for small businesses when considering whether to provide health insurance benefits. The first is Cost. The cost of the premiums to the employer and the employee, and the cost of time in administering the program.

The second is Choice. Can the small employer provide coverage that the employees need, with networks that are sufficient, and out-of-pocket costs that are reasonable?

Again, thank you for holding this roundtable and for inviting me to testify. I look forward to your questions.

Senator ENZI. Thank you.

Mr. Hudak.

STATEMENT OF WARREN S. HUDAK, JR., PRESIDENT, HUDAK AND COMPANY, NEW CUMBERLAND, PA

Mr. HUDAK. Chairman Enzi and members of the Senate HELP Subcommittee on Primary Health and Aging, thank you for the op portunity to be before you today. My name is Warren Hudak. I own a central Pennsylvania based accounting firm. We specialize in bookkeeping, sales tax services, payroll, and tax representation.

Our business is a typical small business. Hudak and Company is a growing firm. But rising healthcare costs continue to consume an increasingly significant share of our revenue. It's difficult to keep up with the constant implementation changes which can disrupt our business operations and consume increasingly more and more of our time. These changes are sometimes meant to help, but occur too late to provide substantial relief. I feel like most small businesses have been placed in an impossible situation. Healthcare costs are once again our No. 1 issue.

Our business has always provided assistance to our employees for health insurance. Group health insurance was expensive and volatile for our business, but we had to offer it in order to compete. We live in the Harrisburg area, which is the State's capital, and we're competing for the same labor market that the State of Pennsylvania is competing for.

We were early adopters of highdeductible group health plans paired with a health savings accounts. Our plan was canceled. We began offering health reimbursement agreements for employees to purchase health insurance on their own. The arrangement worked well for our employees, as they could choose the appropriate plans that fit their needs, even pre existing conditions existed.

I have long been a supporter of those consumerbased options and believe they are key to curbing unsustainable healthcare costs. I, too, believe that the answer here is flexibility and choice.

[The prepared statement of Mr. Hudak follows:]

Prepared Statement of Warren S. Hudak, Jr.

Chairman Enzi, Ranking Member Sanders, and members of the Senate HELP Subcommittee on Primary Health and Retirement Security, thank you for the opportunity to testify before you today concerning rising small business health care costs and potential options for employers and employees to mitigate these cost increases. My name is Warren Hudak, president of Hudak and Company, a central Pennsylvania-based small business accounting firm specializing in payroll services, bookkeeping, sales tax services, and advanced tax transaction analysis.

Our business is a typical small business in many ways. Hudak and Company is a growing firm, but rising health care expenses consume an increasingly significant share of our revenue. It is difficult to keep up with the constant implementation changes, which can be disruptive to our business. These changes are sometimes meant to help, but occur too late to provide substantial relief. I feel like small businesses have been placed in an impossible situation as costs increase and competition and flexibility decrease.

Costs and Limitations

Our business has always provided financial assistance to our employees for health insurance. Group health insurance was expensive and volatile for our business, but we had to offer it in order to compete with larger companies and the Pennsylvania State Government.

We were early adopters to a highdeductible group health plan paired with a health savings account (HSA). Our plan was canceled three different times, so we began offering a health reimbursement arrangement (HRA) for employees to purchase health insurance on their own. The arrangement worked well for our employees as they could choose the appropriate plans that fit their needs, even those with preexisting conditions. I have long been a supporter of consumer-driven health insurance arrangements, and believe they are key to curbing unsustainable health care cost increases.

In 2013, the Internal Revenue Service (IRS) issued guidance[1] that prohibited the use of employer payment plans, including standalone HRAs. Enforcement of the prohibition began July 1, 2015. Facing a threat of $100 per employee per day penalties, we had to again change how we help employees. Any financial assistance must be treated as taxable income, decreasing the value of the contribution, and the contribution cannot be contingent on the purchase of health insurance. It felt like another punch in the nose.

Our family's most recent individual policy premiums increased substantially this year. We shopped around but there was only one other carrier available in our county, and it excluded some of our current doctors, so we stuck with our current plan. Insurance company competition has not improved, it feels worse. It amazes me that there are not more choices in the area. Prescriptions costs have skyrocketed, as well. Costs went up, but coverage worsened.

Options for Relief

I do feel there are policy solutions that can provide relief from high costs for small businesses, provide increased options for small business employees, and provide increased competition amongst insurance companies.

Last week, the House of Representatives passed *the Small Business Health Care Relief Act of 2016* by voice vote.[2] The Senate should quickly consider the bipartisan companion bill.[3] This bill would help employees afford health insurance, and allow employers to continue to play a role in

---

[1] Notice 2013–54, Application of Market Reform and other Provisions of the Affordable Care Act to HRAs, Health FSAs, and Certain other Employer Healthcare Arrangements, *https://www.irs.gov/pub/irs drop/n 13 54.pdf*, (subsequent guidance included in Notice 2015–17).

[2] H.R. 5447, *the Small Business Health Care Relief Act of 2016*, introduced by Congressmen Boustany (RLA) and Thompson (DCA), *https://www.Congress.gov/114/bills/hr5447/BILLS 114hr5447pcs.pdf*, passed on 06/21/2016 (previous version was H.R. 2911).

[3] S. 3060, *the Small Business Health Care Relief Act of 2016*, introduced by Senators Grassley (R IA) and Heitkamp (D ND), *https://www.Congress.gov/114/bills/s3060/BILLS 114s3060 is.pdf*, (previous version was S. 1697).

supporting their employees through the utilization of HRAs. Certainly, lawmakers who drafted the ACA did not intend to punish small businesses for helping their employees with health care costs. Our business is proof that this arrangement worked.

In order to increase competition in my area and other places with limited options, interstate purchasing of insurance plans should be permitted. Interstate purchasing would allow new entrants into markets and force insurance companies to compete for small business and individual customers.

Initial 2017 premium filings in Pennsylvania are discouraging, as insurance companies are requesting significant increases for individual market plans and moderate increases for small business plans. According to NFIB Research Foundation, small business owner optimism remains near historic lows.[4] The political climate continued to be the second most frequently cited reason for why owners think the current period is a bad time to expand. The Senate can begin to restore much needed confidence by quickly sending *the Small Business Health Care Relief Act* to President Obama's desk, and working toward other solutions to lower the cost of health insurance.

Thank you again for allowing me to share small business concerns before the committee today. I look forward to answering any questions.

Senator ENZI. Thank you.

Mr. Harte.

STATEMENT OF THOMAS M. HARTE, PRESIDENT, LANDMARK BENEFITS, INC., HAMPSTEAD, NH

Mr. HARTE. Chairman Enzi, good morning. Ranking Member Sanders, thank you.

---

4 *Small Business Economic Trends*, NFIB Research Foundation, May 2016, *http://www.nfib.com/surveys/small business economic trends/.*

Members of the subcommittee, thank you for having me back again to discuss some of the challenges that are being faced by all of my clients as it relates to health insurance premiums, access to care, access to plans, bifurcated networks, and the many challenges that small businesses are facing in the wake of healthcare reform. As you mentioned in your opening remarks, Senator Enzi, I own an agency back in New Hampshire called Landmark Benefits. I have a bit of a unique position in conversation with you today, because not only am I an employee benefit broker representing thousands of brokers across the country who work tirelessly every single day in advocating for lower premiums for our clients, but also I'm a small business owner.

I have 17 employees, a lot of employees, just like you had back in Wyoming, and I struggle with trying to make sure that they can afford their health insurance premiums for their families, that I can afford to be generous to them. But I sit in that seat of that employer every single day that's faced with these significant rate increases.

I'm also here representing the National Association of Health Underwriters. We represent approximately 100,000 employee benefit professionals across the country. I had the honor of being their national president 2 years ago and served on their board of trustees for a time period of approximately 10 years.

Before I go into some of my comments about some of the challenges that we're faced with, last year, when I was here, I shared with you some of the issues that we needed to face as it relates to affordability, and I wanted to share some positive comments first. First, we have talked about the PACE Act, and, Senator Scott, thank you so much for your sponsorship of that bill and your leadership with Senator Shaheen. It has certainly made a difference in my home State, but has also made a difference in many States across the country.

What my concern was when we were discussing the PACE Act was this concept of what's called rate grid overload, where small employers have these rate grids that are three columns wide, and you can have one family paying $3,000 to $4,000 a month in premium and another family paying $1,500 a month in premium. The invoices are four to five pages long, and it's impossible for small business to manage that process. So I'm grateful, Senator Scott and Senator Shaheen, and thank you for that.

I also am very pleased to share with you that the moratorium on the medical device tax, the delay of the excise tax to 2020, and the health insurance tax suspension for 2017 has been received with open arms in the marketplace, because it's all about affordability. As I may say later, my guiding light is always "Are decisions that we make leading to the accessibility and affordability of health insurance?" I say that to you as Members of Congress, but I also ask that question back home when I'm talking to the health insurance plans.

Now back to the real world of what my clients are facing. Even though we've made some improvements over the past year, I am still delivering rate increases to my clients that are difficult for me to communicate to them, but even more for them to absorb those cost increases. In the past couple of weeks, I have delivered to two clients, who are small businesses, rate increases of 29.96 percent. In my prepared testimony, you will see other clients who are faced with significant doubledigit rate increases.

That contradicts recent trend reports that you've seen in national publications where we're seeing healthcare trends has come down, which is a positive step and a step in the right direction. However, when you have wage growth far below the cost of healthcare, when you have the cost of goods and services across the country rising at a slower rate than healthcare inflation, then we have to ask ourselves the question of how can we really start addressing the underlying issue in our health insurance premiums, which is the cost of healthcare.

I also want to share with you—and I'm sure my friend to my right has faced—when he looks at his own health insurance plan, he has seen that the health insurance companies are making mandatory changes to their plans without the discretion of the employer. Primary care office copays are doubling. Specialist office copays are doubling. Many people across this country are paying upwards of $500 a month for a 30-day supply for a prescription. That's unaffordable, and what's happening is that individuals are foregoing necessary medical treatment and prescriptions to make sure that they can live a healthy life, and that's not what we want. The bottom line for me is in order for us to address the affordability of health insurance, health plans are eliminating plan benefits for individuals. That was never the intent of the Affordable Care Act.

Two more quick issues for you is the recent success that we've seen about the adult uninsured rate dropping—again, good news for the United States of America. However, we have more and more people falling into the category that we commonly refer to as the underinsured. Deductibles have gone through the roof. They've actually increased by 47 percent in recent years, and many employers are purchasing plans that have $5,000 or $6,000 deductibles. Individuals couldn't afford $1,000 deductible, let alone a $5,000 deductible.

The State of Wyoming is not alone. Your home State is not alone. Losing carriers, lack of access to healthcare plans is a growing concern. As a matter of fact, this week, in the State of Minnesota, the largest individual health insurance company, Blue Cross and Blue Shield of Minnesota, announced that they will be exiting the individual marketplace in 2017. So you're not alone.

With that being said, I thank you again for having me back, and I look forward to sharing some other insights with you.

[The prepared statement of Mr. Harte follows:]

Prepared Statement of Thomas M. Harte

Good afternoon. My name is Tom Harte and I am the president of Landmark Benefits Inc. in Hampstead, NH. I started my small business in 1997 and it has become one of the largest independent employee benefit companies in New Hampshire. Today, my company provides services to over 300 corporate clients and the majority are small to midsized businesses. Our primary goal for clients is to provide innovative solutions that address the continued increases in premiums by emphasizing both healthcare quality and healthcare cost containment.

I am proud to be here today on behalf of my professional association, the National Association of Health Underwriters (NAHU), which represents approximately 100,000 health insurance agents, brokers, general agents, consultants and other employee benefit specialists nationally. Last year, I completed 6 years of service as a member of our national Board of Trustees, including serving as the NAHU's national president for 2013–14. As an association member engaged on the national level since 1996, I know thousands of brokers from all over the United States who serve small businesses with health insurance challenges. Not only did I consult with my own clients about their most critical challenges and opportunities with small group coverage that they have asked me to communicate at today's roundtable, but I also reached out to my colleagues nationwide so that I could share their message today.

Prior to my responding to the primary topics for the consideration of the subcommittee, I want to share with you some of the successes within the market since my last visit in July 2015.

- The passing of PACE allowed States to determine if increasing the definition of small group to 100 was in the best interest of their small businesses.
- Delay of Excise Tax to 2020 (Thresholds: $10,200 / $27,500).
- To address the affordability issues in the market, both the Moratorium on Medical Device Tax of 2.3 percent and health insurance tax were suspended for 2017.
- Gallop has reported that the adult uninsured is at 11.0 percent, which is the lowest it has been in 8 years. (*http://www.gallup.com/poll/190484/uninsuredratelowesteight yeartrend.aspx*).

At the same time, it is important to share with you that small businesses continue to face significant premium increases.

Client Location	Enrolled	Deductible	Rate Adj. (In percent)
Manchester, NH	65	$5,000	29.96
Nashua, NH	46	$5,000	29.96
Kittery, ME—SHOP	12	$2,600 HDHP	12.61
Client Location	Enrolled	Deductible	Rate Adj. (In percent)
Lowell, MA.	2	$2,000	29.22
Derry, NH	86	$5,000	18.45
Salem, NH.	10	$500	11.47
Cambridge, MA	19	$2,000	17.73
Methuen, MA.	8	$2,000	15.47
Chelmsford, MA.	3	$2,000	19.01

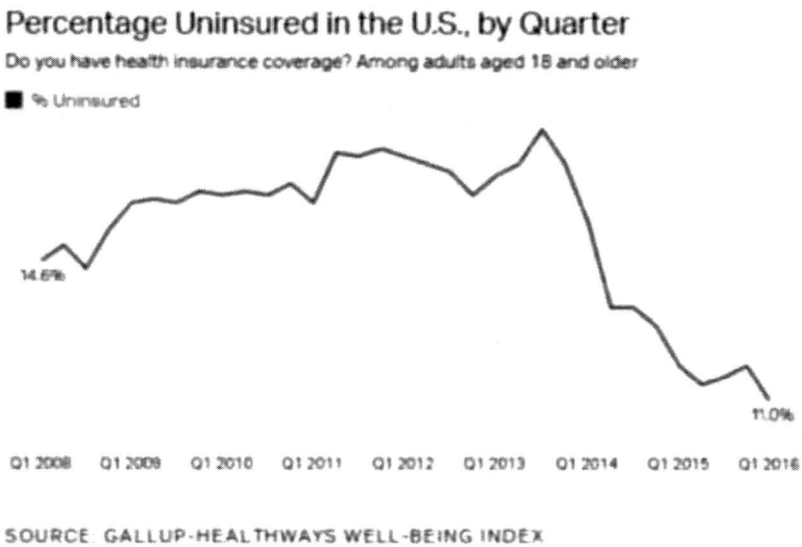

It is also important to understand that most small employers are faced with *mandatory* health plan changes from the health plans. For example:

- Primary care office copays are increasing from $25 to $30 or $40;
- Specialist office copays are increasing from $50 to $60 or $80; and
- Prescription drug copays are increasing dramatically and cost shares are increasing up to a monthly maximum of $400.

Finally, the recent success of the adult uninsured rate at 11.0 percent does not take into consideration the "*under insured*." For example, most employers are increasing plan deductibles and many have increased to as high as $5,000 or $6,000; however, most employees can't afford a deductible event of $1,000 let alone $5,000 or $6,000—this would result in a financial catastrophe.

With regard to the topics of interest to the subcommittee, I have focused my remaining remarks on these issues:

Factors driving healthcare costs for small businesses;

Health insurance market policies that have affected premiums for small businesses; and Factors that small businesses must consider when assisting their employees in purchasing health insurance.

It is my and NAHU's hope that now, 6 years into the implementation of the Patient Protection and Affordable Care Act (ACA), that Congress and President Obama will come together with bipartisan solutions to improve the outcomes of the ACA and resolve many of the unintended consequences that are making coverage more expensive and creating burdens for health insurance consumers.

Factors Driving Healthcare Costs and Health Insurance Market Policies That Have Affected Premiums for Small Businesses

The leading causes of increased health plan premiums are increased utilization and government regulation.

Increased Utilization

In 2014, utilization increased in virtually every metric, with more physician visits, hospitalizations, and prescriptions filled than in 2013. Prior to the recession, higher utilization of services accounted for 43 percent of the increase, fueled by factors such as increased consumer demand, new and more intensive medical treatments, defensive medicine, our aging population, and unhealthy lifestyles. As American consumers return to increasing use of healthcare services, including many newly in sured individuals under the ACA, utilization has increased significantly.

Changes in the rate of utilization could also be attributed to plan design and the use of technologies in place of traditional medicine. To help offset the impact of increasing premiums, insurers and plan administrators have increasingly turned to higher deductibles. From 2009 to 2014, premiums increased by 26 percent in employer sponsored plans while deductibles increased by 47 percent. In 2006, only 10 percent of employers offered plans with deductibles over $1,000 and 3 percent had deductibles over $2,000, compared to 40 percent and 18 percent in 2014, respectively.

Deductible Expenses	X > $1,000	X > $2,000
2006	10 percent of employers	3 percent of employers
2014	40 percent.	18 percent

This increased out-of-pocket expense before coverage is deterring many individuals from seeking necessary healthcare services. This delay of care will exacerbate medical conditions, requiring more expensive care at a later date. Telemedicine is a way that some patients are seeking care without receiving more expensive care in person, as these services can be available at a significantly reduced first-dollar cost to the patient. Other plan design changes include valuebased insurance design, which encourage chronic disease management while reducing the need for more expensive care.

Government Regulation

The ACA has imposed significant compliance burdens on employers, employees, individuals, and local and State government. Many of these compliance burdens discourage employer-sponsored coverage by adding onerous requirements and responsibilities that must be performed on behalf of employees. For small employers, many of the ACA's arbitrary provisions, such as narrow rating bands, limits on composite rating, new levels of minimum coverage, and employer reporting requirements, have resulted in higher costs. However, the compliance burden does not end with just employers, as individuals, providers, State and local governments, and all other elements of the healthcare delivery and financing system must meet the requirements of the law.

On June 14, 2016, the House Energy & Commerce Health Subcommittee held a hearing on "*Advancing Patient Solutions for Lower Costs and Better Care*," which included a discussion of the age rating bands. The age rating bands require insurers to charge their older policyholders three times that of younger policyholders while older policyholders tend to use up to six times as much healthcare in dollar value. This current 3:1 age band rating is a change from what was in effect in the States prior to the ACA when States were able to select their own age band rating, with the most commonly used rating being 5:1. The shift in age rating bands to 3:1 caused an increase in cost to younger policyholders, many of whom would rather drop coverage than pay the increase in premium; however, these are the same group of young, healthy policyholders that are needed in the market in order to avoid adverse selection. I believe that the policy in place prior to the ACA, which allowed States to determine the appropriate age rating bands to implement within their borders, is a far better way to control costs, and in the absence of State action, requiring a 5:1 age band rating would encourage young, healthy policyholders to maintain their coverage and support a far more sustainable health insurance market.

Further, final regulations concerning employer reporting have also burdened employers of all sizes. I can testify that some of my employer clients have spent 100's of hours in preparation, coordination, and deployment of these reporting demands. Additionally, the cost for reporting with either a payroll company or thirdparty administrator is excessive at best. In March 2014, the Department of the Treasury and the Internal Revenue Service (IRS) released final regulations on what health plan information all employers will be required to report to the Federal Government annually for enforcement of both the health reform law's individual and employer mandates. Unfortunately, the final regulations are confusing and extremely complicated for businesses of all sizes. I am concerned that many employers may stop offering health insurance coverage to their employees, especially small employers that are not mandated to do so, because the reporting compliance burden is too much for their business to bear.

There is legislation pending (H.R. 2712 and S. 1996) that will ease the compliance reporting requirements for employers offering health insurance coverage to their employees. The bill clarifies that any information regarding health insurance that is communicated to employees must be aligned with the processes that are already in place by employer or employee, including the use of electronic notification for all notification forms. We believe that providing employees with multiple and similar notices is confusing for employees and both costly and confusing to employers.

Finally, the legislation requires that the Department of the Treasury, in consultation with the Department of Health and Human Services (HHS), Department of Labor, and Small Business Administration, write a report to Congress that would detail the processes necessary to develop a prospective reporting system. Greater sharing of employer plan information between the IRS and HHS to improve exchange subsidy eligibility determinations would work best if the Administration would also allow greater employer flexibility to provide information to employees and health exchanges regarding the employer health coverage offered on a prospective basis. Under a voluntarily prospective reporting system, employers could provide to the IRS information about coverage offered to employees electronically at the employer's openenrollment period or by the January 31 statutory deadline at the employer's election. I believe if greater flexibility was provided and prospective reporting allowed, it will result in greater coordination between the exchanges and the IRS, leading to fewer faulty subsidy determinations and penalty assessments, which, in the long term, will aid in deterring the steady increase of premium costs.

Factors That Small Businesses Must Consider When Assisting Their Employees in Purchasing Health Insurance

It is no surprise that one of the leading factors in considering the purchase of health insurance is cost: cost to both the employee and to the employer. When I spoke to this subcommittee's roundtable last year, I spoke about the dangers of implementing the Cadillac tax. In contrast, today, I am going to shift to address a tax benefit that is in jeopardy, and I would like to take this opportunity to encourage the committee's support for the continuation of the "employer exclusion."

The employer exclusion is used to reference the tax benefit that excludes employer-provided contributions toward an employee's health insurance from that employee's compensation for income and payroll tax purposes. This exclusion makes employer-provided health coverage an attractive form of compensation for workers. According to a new poll from Accenture, three-quarters of workers see health benefits as a "*vital reason*" for continuing to work for their employers, and one-third would quit if their employers stopped offering insurance. A similar percentage said they wouldn't work as hard if their benefits disappeared.

Employer-sponsored coverage is the bedrock of private insurance coverage in the United States. According to the Bureau of Labor Statistics, about 175 million Americans have employer-sponsored coverage and are statistically more likely to maintain coverage year after year. Providing coverage through employers or other group arrangements offers controlled entry and exit in the health insurance market, which ensures the spreading of risk, federally guaranteed consumer protections, like portability rights, the ease of group purchasing and enrollment, and the economies of scale of group purchasing power. In addition, it is a means for employers to provide equitable contributions for their employees.

Several recent health insurance and tax-reform proposals have suggested eliminating or capping the tax exclusion provided to individuals who have employer-provided group coverage and perhaps substituting it for some other tax preference. Capping the exclusion for employees would degrade the benefit and serve as a tax increase for middle-class Americans.

Eliminating the exclusion would mean that most of the advantages of employer-provided coverage would no longer exist: No longer would there be a potent means for spreading risk among healthy and unhealthy individuals; employers and individuals would lose many group purchasing efficiencies; workers would be less likely to have their employer as an advocate in coverage disputes; employers would be less likely to involve themselves in matters of quality assessment and innovation; and employers could suffer in terms of worker productivity and labor costs because employer-sponsored insurance leads far more workers to purchase health insurance than they would on their own. Some employers would not meet participation requirements for group coverage so the entire workforce would lose employer-sponsored coverage. This shift might seem minor, but it could compel employers to stop providing health insurance, according to the Congressional Budget Office and the Joint Committee on Taxation. Companies will expect their employees to secure affordable coverage in the individual market. For many people, particularly older and lower income workers, that may be impossible, even with the implementation of the ACA.

One plan would eliminate the tax exclusion for employer-provided health insurance, preventing companies from purchasing coverage with pre tax dollars, and instead provides individuals with a tax deduction of $7,500 a year for buying insurance. Families would receive a deduction worth $20,500. These types of tax deductions would encourage young, healthy workers to forgo employer-sponsored insurance because they could purchase cheaper plans elsewhere. Employers would be left with an older, sicker risk pool, thus higher costs—if they can get group coverage at all. As costs escalate, even the most generous employers may quit offering health insurance altogether. Delinking coverage from employment like this would make health insurance more expensive and less accessible, thereby contradicting the objectives of the ACA.

Adding to the threat to employer-sponsored insurance is the increase in cost to the employers. In a recent survey, almost 90 percent of businesses reported that their costs had increased because of the law. Employers are responding by laying off workers, making full-time employees part-time so the mandate doesn't apply or dropping coverage altogether. In all three cases, the result is fewer people with employer coverage.

Getting businesses out of the healthcare business would be a mistake. We urge you to maintain the system that has worked for Americans for decades, and preserve employer-sponsored health coverage through the continuation of the employer exclusion.

Small Group Market Policy Recommendations

We all have a stake in having a functioning, viable health insurance marketplace for small employers. While the ACA has brought many changes and market resources to consumers and employers, I am concerned about policies threatening the small group's viability that could lead to its erosion. The membership of the National Association of Health Underwriters feel that the following policy changes would have a significant impact on improving the cost and coverage options available today for our Nation's small employers and their employees:

- To address the affordability of health insurance we need:
  - Further delays of the Excise tax;
  - Continued suspension of the health insurance tax;
  - Continued moratorium on medical device tax; and
  - Legislation that allows States to increase the law's age rating bands from the current 3:1 spread to bands that more closely resembles the natural breakdown of age and meet the needs of a particular State. If a State does not set its own bands, the default should be 5:1.
- Preservation of the law's risk-adjustment mechanisms (often referred to as "The Three Rs") since they are crucial to preserving long-term private insurance market stability.
- To address the accessibility of health insurance we need:
  - To remove agent and broker commissions from the medical loss ratio calculation in the small and individual health insurance markets, to ensure small business access to agent

and broker services and to economically help the hundreds of thousands of agent small business owners nationwide.

- To address the simplification of health insurance we need:
  - A repeal of the employer mandate, or failing, that establishes the eligibility threshold at 101 or more employees; and
  - To allow employers to set the definition of a full-time employee as one that works 40 or more hours a week for health coverage purposes.

In closing, I would like to thank Chairman Enzi, Ranking Member Sanders and all of the members of the subcommittee for the amazing opportunity to share information about the opportunities and challenges small business owners like me and my clients are having in today's health insurance marketplace. If you have any questions or need more information, please do not hesitate to contact me at either (603) 329–4535 or *tharte@landmarkbenefits.com*.

Senator ENZI. Thank you.

Ms. Lueck.

STATEMENT OF SARAH LUECK, SENIOR POLICY ANALYST, CENTER ON BUDGET AND POLICY PRIORITIES, WASHINGTON, DC

Ms. LUECK. Thank you, Mr. Chairman, and thank you, members of the subcommittee, for having me here today. I really appreciate the opportunity to talk about issues facing small businesses with their healthcare.

As my other copanelists have mentioned, there are longstanding systemwide trends in healthcare costs that absolutely affect small businesses, and that's a key question, obviously, one that we'll be discussing as we get into the conversation here today. As has been widely documented, also, the overall healthcare cost growth has slowed considerably in recent years with health reform likely a key contributor. While we don't have all the answers, we certainly appear to be making some improvements in bending that cost curve. Another piece of good news is that contrary to predictions, the ACA hasn't caused employers to drop coverage for their workers so far, and that's really good news. I'm impressed to hear those small business owners that are on this panel talking about how important it is to offer benefits. It's nice to hear the commitment that they have to their employees and the variety of considerations they make when they decide whether to offer benefits and what kind of benefits to offer.

As somebody who focuses a lot on the ACA and supports so many of the provisions that were in that law, I really wanted to mention the way in which the coverage expansions under the ACA have actually helped small businesses, the employees of those small businesses, by making sure that they have access to coverage and can maintain their health regardless of whether a small employer that they work for is able to offer them coverage. That's very important, if they're a lowwage worker, that they have access to Medicaid in a State that has taken up the coverage expansion and that they can also access subsidized coverage through the marketplace, where they both get assistance with affording the coverage and then reductions in the high deductibles and other costsharing so that they can also have some access to healthcare.

Notably, many selfemployed people have also newly obtained in surance as a result of the ACA, and it's just worth thinking about—the situations that people used to face before the law was in place. Self employed people might have had trouble getting access to coverage if they had a preexisting health condition, and now they can get access to coverage in the individual market.

The essential health benefits were mentioned as something that was sort of bad news. In some ways, I think, for many people, it's good news to have some minimum standards about the benefits that are covered under small group plans. Before the ACA, there might have been gaps in the coverage that small employers were able to choose from in their State. Their employees, just like individuals that don't have employer coverage, want access to maternity benefits, for example, or mental health treatments, and those sorts of things may not have been covered in their policies before in some cases.

Another story we used to hear before the law was in place is those cases where a small business might have a sick employee, somebody diagnosed with a very expensive illness or an employee who has a baby that's born with a lot of challenging health problems and has to be hospitalized. Those sorts of huge costs that one person in a small firm could face could really impact the cost of coverage for that small business just the following year.

That might put a small firm, a small business owner, in the position of thinking, "Can I even offer coverage now that I have this expensive claim on my books?" That is not an issue now under the ACA. There's broader pooling and limits on the way that the insurers can rate small groups, just as there are with the rules in the individual market.

I think with that, I'll pause. I'll just say, also, that there's a lot of good news here. I think that there's a lot of flexibility, also, for

States that want to take some opportunities to do things in their own markets to stabilize it, to make things more competitive, and, hopefully, we will get into some of those issues as we continue our discussion today.

Thank you very much.

[The prepared statement of Ms. Lueck follows:]

Prepared Statement of Sarah Lueck

Chairman Enzi and Ranking Member Sanders, thank you for the opportunity to discuss the challenges and opportunities for small businesses that want to provide health benefits to their workers.

What Factors Are Driving Health Care Costs For Small Businesses?

Longstanding systemwide trends in health care costs and utilization affect all health care payers, including small employers that offer health insurance to their workers. For example, the entry of highcost specialty drugs into the market can raise premiums for small businesses and the workers they cover. Other trends, however, can slow growth in health care costs and premiums, including adoption of new payment models that encourage the use of highvalue services and efforts to increase competition among insurers based on price and quality of care.

As has been widely documented, overall health care cost growth has slowed considerably in recent years, with health reform likely a key contributor. Premium increases for employers have been similarly modest in most States since the Affordable Care Act's (ACA) enactment; average jobbased premiums rose only 4 percent between 2014 and 2015. Premiums between 2010 and 2015 rose 27 percent, which was significantly lower than the 69 percent increase from 2000 to 2005.[5] There has been, however, a long-term trend toward workers paying a growing share of premiums and cost-sharing charges under employer-sponsored plans. For example, annual deductibles continue to rise, and more workers are enrolled in plans that include deductibles.

Contrary to predictions, the ACA hasn't caused employers to drop coverage for their workers. From 2014 to 2015, the percentage of employees who reported that their employers offer health coverage increased slightly, as did the share who reported being eligible for the coverage offered, according to a new analysis of Census data. Overall coverage rates remained stable for people working at both small and large employers during that period.[6]

Smaller employers remain less likely than larger ones to offer coverage, however. In fact, the smaller the firm, the less likely it offers coverage. For example, in 2015, 37 percent of firms with three to nine workers reported offering coverage, as compared to 63 percent of firms with 10 to 24 workers, 82 percent of firms with 25 to 49 workers, and 92

---

[5] Kaiser Family Foundation and Health Research & Educational Trust, "*Employer Health Ben efits 2015 Annual Survey*," September 2015.

[6] Joelle Abramowitz and Brett O'Hara, "New Estimates of Offer and Take up of Employer Sponsored Insurance," June 2016, forthcoming publication in *Medical Care Research & Review*.

percent of firms with 50 to 199 workers. Firms that do not offer health benefits cite cost as the main reason.[7]

The ACA's coverage expansions have undoubtedly helped small business employees by ensuring that more people have access to coverage through Medicaid and the marketplaces. Many small business employees and their family members who may have been uninsured in the past can receive needed medical care and maintain their health. Notably, many self-employed people have also newly obtained insurance as a result of the ACA. Self-employed people often could not get coverage before the ACA, when insurers in most States' individual markets could deny coverage or charge far higher rates based on preexisting health conditions. For example, more than one-fifth of the enrollees in California's individual market exchange (known as Covered California) were selfemployed as of June 2016.[8]

What Federal Insurance Market Policies Have Affected Premiums for Small Businesses?

Federal policies under the ACA have produced a much better functioning small group market than existed prior to health reform. Some of these policies have enabled small employers to improve the coverage they offer, while others have lowered premiums, particularly for firms with older workforces in poorer health.

Insurers offering coverage in the small group market must now cover a package of "essential health benefits," which includes critical benefits like maternity services and treatment for mental health and substance abuse disorders; before health reform, these benefits were often omitted from small group plans, even if small employers wanted to offer them. The ACA also bans annual and lifetime dollar limits on the benefits that insurers pay out and requires plans to limit enrollees' out-of-pocket costs each year for deductibles, copayments, and other cost sharing charges. While these reforms made small group coverage more comprehensive and hence pushed up premiums somewhat, they also enabled small firms to offer

---

[7] Kaiser Family Foundation and Health Research Educational Trust, *op cit*.

[8] Covered California data is available upon request.

coverage more similar to the offerings from large employers, a choice that many small firms did not have before the ACA.

Other Federal policy changes affect how insurers set premiums for the small group market, including a prohibition on charging higher premiums based on employees' health status, gender, industry type, or the overall claims history of a small business, as well as a limit on how much more insurers can charge older employees than younger ones. While some small businesses have seen premium increases due to these changes (for example, those whose workers are mostly younger, healthier, or male), other firms have seen premium decreases (for example, those whose work ers are mostly older, sicker, or female). As a result, all small employers covered by ACA compliant policies, including those with younger and healthier workers, can rest easier now that a sudden illness among their workers or their workers' families will not result in a sudden spike in the firm's premiums the following year, which was a substantial risk for small businesses prior to 2014.

The ACA also requires each insurer in the small group market to pool their enrollees in that market when determining what they will charge for coverage. Advocates for small businesses have long wanted the ability to pool small firms together to get more affordable and stable premiums, similar to large employers, rather than having each small firm looked at independently when setting premiums. Broader pooling, too, has allowed some firms to see their rates decrease or to stay the same. Other firms (such as those with healthier and younger workers) may have seen higher premiums as a result, but in the long run, premiums in the small group mar ket will likely be more stable over time due to this single risk pool requirement than they would otherwise have been.

The ACA also required insurers in the individual and small group markets to spend 80 percent of the premiums they charge on patient care and quality improvement efforts. Prior to health reform, only about 70 percent of insurers in the small group market met this "medical loss ratio" (MLR) standard, which means that more than 20 percent of small business premiums were going to overhead and profit rather than medical care. The MLR requirement helps ensure that small businesses get good value for their premium contributions. In addition, ACA mandated improvements in information transparency for small businesses make it far easier for busi ness owners to compare plan and coverage options. For example, a standard form called a Summary of Benefits and Coverage (SBC) allows apples-to-apples comparison of virtually any plan's benefits and cost sharing charges. The ACA's standards for plan benefits and cost sharing charges, including the "metal levels" that small group plans must meet, also help consumers compare coverage options, promoting competition based on price and quality among insurers—which can help reduce premiums.

While health reform established some minimum Federal standards for State small group markets, States remain primarily responsible for their markets. States have a number of tools to improve affordability for small businesses (as well as individuals) and create more affordable, competitive, and stable markets. For example, States that have the authority to review and either approve or disapprove health insurers' proposed rates have helped reduce premium increases compared to what insurers wanted to charge. Some States operate Small Business Health Options Program (or SHOP) marketplaces, which offer a choice of plans and carriers to small business employees and allow some small employers to receive Federal tax credits for offering coverage.

A few States have taken additional steps to ensure that their risk pools are well-balanced and as competitive as possible. For example, Vermont and Massachusetts each merged their individual and small group markets. Vermont includes small businesses with up to 100 employees in its merged market, rather than up to 50 employees as in most States.

Many States also decided not to extend the availability of non ACA compliant plans for small businesses. In States that allowed such plans to continue (under an Administration policy), some degree of adverse selection likely occurred that weakened the stability of the small group market. Firms with healthier workers are likely disproportionately enrolled in those plans. States that did not continue to make those plans available likely helped create more balanced risk pools more quickly in their small group markets, with more stable premiums.

What Factors Must Small Businesses Consider When Assisting Employees In Purchasing Health Insurance?

Small employers have a number of options for assisting workers with purchasing insurance. The first question is whether to offer health benefits at all, if the employer is small enough to be exempt from the "shared responsibility" penalty. Clearly, many small employers view health benefits as critical to attracting and retaining highquality workers and will continue offering them even if not required to. Other small firms may decide not to offer health coverage, recognizing that the reformed individual market is far more accessible due to the ACA. Workers and their family members with preexisting health conditions now have guaranteed access to an individual market plan that covers a comprehensive set of benefits and protects against very high out-of-pocket costs.

Many small business employees may also qualify for Federal premium tax credits and costsharing subsidies for coverage purchased through an individual market exchange or marketplace if they are not offered employer-sponsored coverage or the coverage is not affordable or comprehensive.

Another option for small employers is to offer small group health coverage to their workers, possibly by working with an insurer or a broker, much as they did before the ACA. Some may use private exchanges to access small group coverage.

One additional option created by the ACA within the small group market is SHOP, as noted above. SHOP gives small businesses an easier way to comparison shop for insurance options, receive tax credits, and offer multiple plan options to their workers. The SHOP exchanges got off to a slower start than the individual marketplaces and have suffered from some technical and operational problems, so enrollment remains low. However, it appears the technical issues have largely been resolved. In 2016, employee choice—which allows employers to select a metal tier and employees to choose any SHOP plan in that tier—became available in all States served by the federally run SHOP. This was an important advance; previously, small firms typically could offer only one insurance plan from one carrier. In addition to reducing the effort involved with offering coverage, the SHOP enables small businesses that want to contribute to the cost of a small group plan on a tax advantaged basis to do so.

Yet another option in many States—and one that raises significant concerns for the stability of premiums in the small group market—is the possibility that small businesses will increasingly decide to selfinsure, meaning they would bear the risk of employees' medical claims. Some small employers might find this attractive, at least at first, because it would allow them to offer coverage that doesn't meet many of the ACA's requirements for the small group market. Insurers offering to help small employers selfinsure also provide a reinsurance or stoploss policy to cover unexpectedly large claims. However, selfinsurance would most likely attract employers with workers that tend to be healthier and cost less to cover. If a large share of small employers with lower cost employees opt to selfinsure, this would disrupt the newly balanced risk pools in States' small group markets and make premiums less affordable and stable over time.

Finally, the House recently passed a bill allowing firms with fewer than 50 workers to use a health reimbursement arrangement (HRA) to contribute to the cost of workers' premiums on the individual market. Currently such "standalone" HRAs are not permitted because they cannot meet ACA standards for group health plans offered by employers, such as the requirement to cover certain preventive services at no cost and the prohibition against annual benefit limits. Similar to selfinsurance by small groups, standalone HRAs for small employers (which have been banned for all employers since 2014) could have a negative impact on States' small group markets. It is unclear how many small businesses that now offer coverage might shift their workers to the individual market using an HRA and how that might affect workers and the risk pool in a given State. However, large numbers of small firms could decide to make this jump. If they tend to be firms with healthier workers, this could leave the small businesses remaining in the small group market with higher premiums and possibly fewer coverage options.

Supporters of the HRA proposal claim that it would free up more low income workers to get subsidized coverage through the marketplace, rather than requiring them to take an employer offer of coverage that might not be as affordable or comprehensive. But it isn't clear how employers would structure their offers in response to the HRA proposal. Employers have significant flexibility to define the terms of the HRA they offer, and many low-wage workers might not be better off. Such an option, if made available to small employers, seems ill advised because of its risks for the small group market.

Senator ENZI. Thank you.

We'll get into a little discussion. As I mentioned, this is a roundtable, so if somebody wants to make a comment, if you'll stand your name tag up, you can comment on anything that's been said or any of the questions that might come up. Of course, one of the things we're concentrating on here is cost, and I'd be interested in any suggestions that you might have—you may have already stated them—on ways to bring those costs down for small businesses.

Does anybody want to answer that question? Mr. Glause.

Mr. GLAUSE. Thank you, Senator Enzi. One thing we need to focus on is that healthcare determines the cost of health insurance. Health insurance doesn't dictate the cost of healthcare. I think we need to really take a look at how we're going to control our healthcare costs and our pharmacy costs.

When you talk to the health insurance companies, the No. 1 driving factor for increase in rates is continued prescription cost. I think that our discussion, if we're going to really look at focusing on controlling the cost of insurance, has to include looking at the delivery of healthcare.

Senator ENZI. Thank you. Mr. Harte.

Mr. HARTE. I figure I'll be a great segue to Commissioner Glause, because a lot of what we talk about at the Health Underwriters is something that I've been preaching from the rooftops for a very long time, and that is that health insurance is expensive because healthcare is expensive. As a matter of fact, within the ACA, it talked a lot about the medical loss ratios, and we've talked about that issue for years.

When you think about the medical loss ratio from a cost of healthcare perspective, when formulating healthcare reform, when medical loss ratio came out, finally, it came out at 85 percent for large group and 80 percent for small group. That speaks volumes to me about healthcare, because a lot of what we talk about across the country are health insurance premiums, but people are bundling it all together to say that the problem is health insurance premiums.

In fact, when 80 percent to 85 percent of the cost of the premiums goes toward healthcare, a lot of our focus should be more on the healthcare side of the delivery equation. When I reflect back and I look at statistics going back to 2014, when we look at metrics—and we look at metrics as inpatient hospital care, physician visits, hospitalization—since that time, all of those metrics have gone through the roof. As a result, healthcare costs have exploded, which leads to higher health insurance premiums.

Then, of course, like I mentioned before, the deductibles for the individuals are making it unaffordable for them to have access to care. A 47 percent increase in deductibles from 2009 to 2014 makes healthcare unaffordable for a lot of people. Yes, they're insured, and that's what we wanted to do. That's what we wanted to accomplish with accessibility. But in the end, we're making healthcare very unaffordable.

As it relates to prescriptions, what a lot of people don't know is when we talk to an employer, 26 percent to 28 percent of their premium goes toward prescription cost expenses. We tend to set that aside because we're simply paying a $10 or $25 copay. But in the end, we have insureds who have prescriptions that cost $100,000 per month, $100,000 a month for one prescription. We need to address the cost of prescriptions.

Then we move into highcost claimants. Historically, Health Un derwriters—we look at the total healthcare dollar, and it's commonly known that 5 percent of the claimants produce 50 percent of the total utilization of an employer plan. That's a challenge for us, because as a health underwriter myself, as a compassionate individual, I desperately want to make sure that we take care of those people who are suffering from chronic illness. But we need a solution to address the 50 percent of the healthcare equation.

I will yield my time over to Sarah. Ms. Lueck. I think he was next. Mr. Harte. Oh, I'm sorry.

Senator ENZI. Mr. Hudak.

Mr. HUDAK. Fundamental to shaving the cost of care is transparency. Americans are great consumers. We consume better than anybody else. We know how to shop. One could argue under the Affordable Care Act that there's less transparency, not more transparency. There's less options, not more options. In our area, we have three viable options. We are paying $200 a month more for our family coverage just to keep our doctors, to stay in—so that my wife can keep her doctors.

Consumer-based health plans gives the flexibility and allows us to be consumers. I have some stories about being a consumer. When going to the doctor and they see that you have a highdeductible health plan, they'll negotiate the price with you. "Mr. Hudak, if you pay today, we'll give you a 20 percent decrease in the bill."

But it's more than that. It's how I get my care, what care I get. I had to have a procedure done on my back. The doctor deemed it elective. I said, "No, I have a tremendous amount of pain. It's affecting my work. It's affecting my ability to run my business." The doctor said, "I can't justify it with the insurance company." I had an HSA. I said, "I'll pay for it. It's not a big deal." We negotiated our price. I had the procedure done.

In 2 months, I lost 30 pounds, 30 pounds in 2 months. I felt better than I had in a decade. My productivity went up. My business thrived. Today, I need to have the procedure done again. Guess what? They don't want to do it. I don't have the flexibility. I don't have the options I had when I was a consumer. I'd like to be a consumer again.

Senator ENZI. Ms. Lueck.

Ms. LUECK. Thank you. I think one thing I wanted to point out is there is a lot of discussion about consumer-driven healthcare, and I think there are some things, particularly, as you mentioned, related to transparency that can help consumers be better informed. There are now standard forms called SBCs that exist for virtually every plan.

If you are trying to decide what plan you want to buy, whether it's maybe your spouse's plan and yours from two different employers or you're in the marketplace and you're shopping for individual market coverage, you can lay these documents side by side, and this is the first time you've ever been able to compare apples to apples, sort of. What is the cost sharing for this plan versus this plan? Which benefits are excluded? The insurers provide those and the employers provide those for almost every plan. That's a really helpful thing for people to begin to understand their plans and how they work and to try to make wise choices about coverage when they're looking for coverage.

But when it comes to consumer-directed healthcare, I think we're often talking about very highdeductible plans, which, as we've already said, are difficult for people. The problem with a very highdeductible plan is that it can be kind of a blunt instrument that makes the person perhaps decide not to get care and they may not be making the best decision in terms of whether to get high-value care or low-value care. They may just sort of be deciding "I'm not going to get this care because I can't afford my deductible," and that's not something we want to see.

Some of the more sophisticated and perhaps impactful things that are starting to go on, I think, to deal with healthcare costs have to do with driving provider behavior, because providers have a lot of power in the system. When they're dealing with consumers, as the anecdote showed, making decisions about cost and value of care and deciding how to proceed with treatment, often that's something the consumer can't do on their own or can't do enough to make a difference in healthcare costs, because a lot of things either aren't elective for them or they don't have enough information about the specific medical benefits and costs to make a decision or about the prices of the treatment.

I think that we have a lot of work to do. But I think that there's a lot of promise in trying to change payment structures in order to drive higher value care, reduce inefficient care, and to maybe encourage providers to talk with patients about how best to proceed with treatments.

STATEMENT OF SENATOR SCOTT

Senator SCOTT. Mr. Chairman.

Senator ENZI. Tim.

Senator SCOTT. These folks are fairly active with these name tags going up and down, so I figured I'd just jump in here now.

Senator ENZI. Yes.

Senator SCOTT. Thank you.

Senator ENZI. We'll come back to that.

Senator SCOTT. Yes, we certainly will, because I'm going to focus on the issues, because I think if we take a step back and realize what we're having a conversation about, we're having a conversation about healthcare affordability for small businesses, but really for employees of small businesses, for average families, who in the last several years have seen their real income go down, not up. We've seen more small businesses closed last year than opened. There's a reason why.

In the economy that we are facing today, we have 12 million more Americans who are living in poverty. We have a 40 percent increase in Americans who are eligible for food stamps. There's something going wrong in our economy, and if you look at one of the primary challenges we face, especially as a former small business owner for 15 years, the regulatory environment that exists today is unparalleled in the history of our country.

Six of the last 7 years, we've seen the greatest increase in regulatory burden: 80,000 new pages proposed last year with an economic impact of $1.8 trillion. We're asking small businesses to do what they've never had to do before. If you look at two of the primary causes for the regulatory burden that we see today—Dodd Frank and the ACA.

When you focus specifically on the ACA and you ask yourself the question between healthcare costs and health insurance, perhaps it's the wrong debate, because I would tell you that the ACA may actually be increasing the actual cost of healthcare, because what you talked about for a moment there, Mr. Harte, was what I call healthcare rationing. You may have a card that gives you access, but because of providers—and in South Carolina, we've had two rural hospitals closed. Yes, you have a card, but do you have access to healthcare?

With higher deductibles—and we may be talking about HSAs, where your deductible is $5,000. But, actually, in South Carolina and throughout this country, it is difficult for the average American to put $400 together, not $5,000, but $400. We're talking about people working paycheck to paycheck, who are struggling to make a $1,000 deductible or a $500 deductible. In November, we're going to hear about higher health insurance costs, not lower.

Mr. Hudak, who had to negotiate for his healthcare cost because of the challenges of health insurance, may not always be in the position to negotiate again for the necessary back surgery that increases his productivity, not decreases it. I would love for us to continue the conversation on how small employers can better afford to provide healthcare coverage for their employees. But I want to make sure that we do so, looking through the prism of reality.

Anyone who believes that when 12 out of 23 coops fail, 740,000 more folks looking for coverage because of the failure, when the exchanges are challenged, when health insurance coverage is becoming more expensive, and when United Healthcare, one of the largest providers, is saying, "No, I can't do that anymore. I'm pulling out"—for us to think that reducing competition somehow lowers prices, it's only in Washington where that makes sense, to be honest with you.

Mr. Hudak, I do have a few questions for you and Mr. Harte as well, and the panel can answer the questions. I'll start with you, Mr. Hudak.

Sixty percent of small employers suggest—and I would say states—that the reason why they don't have health insurance for their employees 52 percent of the time is because of cost. What are some of the reasons that you've seen, as an accountant, with folks that you're insuring? You're having a lot of interaction with folks financially. What are some of the things that you're hearing from the folks that you work with on the cost issue, if you can answer that question? No. 2, how will increased premiums—we see they're coming in November of this year—impact the number of folks that you think will be providing health insurance in the future?

Then for the panel, I think—and I can't prove this yet—but I think the employer mandate and the penalty will actually create a perverse incentive to provide less healthcare through your employer, not more healthcare—

2,000 versus 10,000 might be an easy conclusion to reach for many employers. The actual burden on taxpayers will go up, not down.

First, healthcare costs from the small business perspective— what have you seen? Mr. Hudak and Mr. Harte as well, I know that you are in the business. I sold health insurance for about 5 years and realized, OMG, I need to do something else. So I went into the property and casualty business and the financial services business.

I see the pain. I've seen the pain that an increase has when someone who could barely afford their health insurance could see doubling of their health insurance costs, even though they have an HSA. In South Carolina, a guy in Greenville went from $425 a month to $800 for his family with a $25,000 deductible, family deductible.

Mr. HUDAK. The small business community has always struggled with healthcare premiums. That's why we always liked the flexibility of consumer-based products. In order to compete with the State of Pennsylvania, because of our proximity to the capital, we provided an HRA, an allowance, allow our employees to have a certain dollar amount that we could afford. We can budget for it. We can plan. We can figure it into our growth plan.

What we found, particularly amongst young people, millennials, is they love that flexibility. They love to be able to take that money—and maybe their wife has a medical plan at her employer, but maybe they don't have dental, or maybe they need help with their copays, or maybe they need help with their coinsurance. This enables us the flexibility to compete for that labor. All big businesses become big businesses with the help of great people, and we need to attract and retain those. Sure, we'd like to provide health insurance.

You asked about what's happening. We have a business on our board, on the NFIB board in Pennsylvania. He had been providing health insurance for 40 years. He was prideful. It was a bragging point. Do you know that last year, he announced that he can no longer afford coverage for his firm anymore, and those individuals ended up in the marketplace? It's unfortunate. It made him less competitive. It made his business, some may argue, less attractive to young talented people that can maybe bring his business to the next level.

What we've found with the Affordable Care Act is we have greater costs. We went from $1,200 a month for our family plan to $1,900, if we include my wife's prescriptions, which went from $100 to $600 a month. When we signed up for the plan, we specifically asked about the formulary for that drug. They assured me—but because of the confusion, even the insurance company got it wrong. We signed up for a plan, and they couldn't even—when we signed up, they didn't truly represent the cost to us. There's not less confusion. There's more confusion.

Senator SCOTT. Mr. Harte.

Mr. HARTE. Thank you. Off testimony, because you were a broker yourself at one time—yes, maybe you were the smart one. You got out after 5 years. I've been doing this for almost 30 years.

Senator SCOTT. Let us pray.

Mr. HARTE. I would say brokers across the country—we struggle every single day. We struggle because those who become our clients become our family. We take them under our wing. We help them every single day, not just with the price increases that they are so fearful of every 12 months, but having access to care and the other challenges with their health insurance plan.

Before I flew down here, I took a sampling of my most recent re newals that I've had, and I gathered 12 of them just so that I can share with you the insights from my employers. It's hard for me to walk into a small business and say, "Your rate has increased by 29.96 percent," or 18.45 percent, 17.73 percent, 15.47 percent. The fact is small businesses have to make a critical decision—How much of this am I going to pass on to my employees? How much of it can I absorb on my own? What must I cut? What type of cost shifting do I need to do? Do I need to reduce my prescriptions, increase the hospital copays? What do I need to do?—because they can't afford a 30 percent rate increase.

As you indicated earlier, with the struggles within our economy, employers are struggling—small, medium, large businesses, and individuals who are purchasing insurance on the marketplace. It's unsustainable for us to continue to be faced with these significant rate increases.

I know we talked briefly about transparency, and I believe transparency is one of the success factors that we really need to focus on. Anecdotally, it always helps me when I share numbers. On my phone, I have this really cool app. It's not available to you, Senator Scott, because you're in South Carolina. But I have this app in New Hampshire. It's called My Medical Shopper, and I can scroll through, and I can find out what the cost is within 30 miles of my home of any particular service that I need, and it's all bundled up. It brings one particular care together.

For your interest, I threw together a couple of examples. I'll give you four, and they were picked at random for me when I was out in New Mexico yesterday. For an MRI of a lumbar spine without dye, the least expensive facility within 30 miles of my home is $485. The most expensive is $2,114. The percentage is 436 percent. Colonoscopy—the least expensive is $458. The most expensive is $3,031. The percentage is 661 percent.

STATEMENT OF SENATOR CASSIDY

Senator CASSIDY. Does that include facility fees?

Mr. HARTE. Yes, it is.

Senator CASSIDY. Is that soup to nuts?

Mr. HARTE. Soup to nuts. This particular app will actually show you all of the other underlying care that happens with that particular colonoscopy. The one that's up on my phone right now is with a biopsy. It can drill down to a very specific and deliberate procedure. The MRI categories that are on this app go into maybe 30 or 40 different categories of MRIs, with dye or not, neck, back, legs, arms.

Senator CASSIDY. Is it the provider who is publishing that, or is it the insurance company which is publishing that rate schedule? Mr. HARTE. For this particular app, they are doing a technology platform called scraping, where they're going in to the back end of the website for the health insurance company and pulling the data from the health insurance company.

Senator CASSIDY. That's pretty cool.

Senator SCOTT. One last question before we hear more on this. One of the things that I think escapes us at times is the impact of the medical loss ratio on a small business person's opportunity to have an expert come in, because, essentially, you're shaving commissions, and, frankly, in a world that's becoming more complicated, you're having fewer experts come in to provide assistance, which makes it more likely that a small business owner will opt out of providing care. Remember that 60 percent of employees work for a company with 20 or fewer employees.

Mr. HARTE. You're talking my language, Senator Scott. So, yes, and within healthcare reform, between small group and large group, the medical loss ratios must be 80 percent or 85 percent, dependent upon where you fall as an employer. Broker compensation must be included within the administrative costs. We have argued for years that that should be pulled out, because there's no greater value to an employer than accessing the expertise of an employee benefit professional who can help small businesses like Mr. Hudak. The fact is purchasing health insurance is not like going down to your appliance store and buying a refrigerator. Purchasing health insurance is overwhelmingly complicated. Whether you talk about deductibles or coinsurance or transparency or bifurcated networks, it is likely the most complicated product that you will ever have to purchase, and you need the expertise of an employee benefit professional to help you navigate those challenges.

Senator SCOTT. Thank you.

Thank you, Mr. Chairman, for your indulgence.

Senator ENZI. Thank you for your questions.

Senator Cassidy, I know, has questions, because he's been working on this a lifetime, and since he's gotten to the Senate, he's spent another lifetime working on it.

Senator CASSIDY. And my hair has turned your color. [Laughter.]

Senator CASSIDY. It used to be, shall we say, blond.

Ms. Lueck, you had a critique of consumer-driven healthcare that their high deductibles make perhaps less advantageous. Oftentimes, I think of consumer-driven healthcare as a health savings account associated with that catastrophic policy. On the other hand, the exchange policies typically have a $6,000 deductible without the HSA component.

Now, it seems as if you're OK with the one, but have kind of a negative critique of the other. How do you reconcile that impression that I have?

Ms. LUECK. On the exchanges, for people who are low-income, who are under 250 percent of the poverty line, there are cost sharing reductions available, and it varies in terms of how that affects the deductible under a Silver Plan, but it can affect it quite significantly. For the people that are lowest income, the deductibles are substantially reduced, and that's important because there's a lot of research to show that lower income people are really sensitive to price, and they would possibly avoid care that they should be getting because they can't afford to pay the fee that they owe.

Senator CASSIDY. Though what we're hearing from Mr. Hudak and others is that, really, a single woman who's earning $70,000 a year would not qualify for a subsidy. Mr. Harte, how much does a single woman in New Hampshire who is 45 years old pay for an individual policy, Silver policy?

Mr. HARTE. Approximately $600 a month.

Senator CASSIDY. She is paying $7,200 a year on a pretax income of $70,000. She's paying probably roughly 15 percent of her after tax income, if not more, and I find that if she has a $6,000 deductible, she also is foregoing care. Again, if you're limiting your comments to those who are getting subsidized, I guess I see your point. If we're going to be more inclusive of the middle class and these people who are typical employees, they're getting punished, and I'm not sure how—they have a $6,000 deductible with a pretax income of—you see where I'm going with that. Any comments on that?

Ms. LUECK. Yes. I mean, I think that we definitely need to look closely at the affordability of cost sharing and how it's impacting people and whether the HSAstyle plan with a high deductible is the best route to go, regardless of your income, and whether people are able to make the decisions about how to spend that money, when, as Senator Scott pointed out, a lot of people have trouble even spending $400 out-of-pocket if they needed to in a pinch.

Another point I should make about the ACA compliant plan design is what we've seen over time. A trend that's different than what was there before in terms of plan design is that, often, even a plan that has a very high deductible of $6,000, like you're mentioning, may cover a lot of services that people commonly use without charging them that deductible.

Senator CASSIDY. It will for a colonoscopy, but it will not for the car accident or the trip to the urgent care center with their daughter's earache, and that is where they are foregoing care, anecdotally, in order to still put food on the table. That seems inherent in the rate structure that is part of the ACA exchanges.

Ms. LUECK. There's a variety of ways that they design plans. When there's a car accident, people aren't able to decide one way or the other, right, and if they don't have the money to pay——

Senator CASSIDY. But they are left with that hanging over them, and although the ACA was supposed to eliminate medical bankruptcy, I gather it is actually a worse problem now. Let me ask as well—sitting here, it's like you're hearing two different conversations.

From you, sir, I heard dramatic increases in premiums, and from you and from you, and then—or at least out-of-pocket exposure and the inability to afford. From Ms. Lueck, I heard from you that premiums are only rising 4 percent. It really is a kind of discordance as we listen.

The way I reconcile that—but tell me if you disagree, Ms. Lueck, because people who defend the ACA mention that 4 percent. But that's not out-of-pocket exposure. That is premium cost. Premium costs may be only rising 4 percent, but network is narrowing and out-of-pocket exposure is increasing. That 4 percent rise means the policy now has a higher deductible, a higher copay, tiered benefits for pharmacies—I could go on.

You're nodding your head, Mr. Harte.

Ms. Lueck, do you agree even though premiums are not rising, that patients' out-of-pocket exposure has increased substantially?

Ms. LUECK. Premiums are rising more slowly in recent years. They're still rising, and I think that's a longstanding trend, obviously. Then there's a longstanding trend toward individuals bearing more of their own out-of-pocket costs compared to the employer in things like deductibles and cost sharing. I don't point at the ACA. That's a trend that predates the ACA, and I think that the key thing that the ACA did is expand coverage for people so there are actually a lot fewer people that are facing the kind of bankruptcy that you're talking about.

Senator CASSIDY. I've seen the statistics. The statistics show that medical bankruptcies have not declined. Imagine a family in a wreck in December—they have complete exposure—then they're in the wreck, so there's still pain through the next year. That's actually an unfulfilled promise, if you will.

Ms. LUECK. We continue to have affordability issues. You mentioned the woman with a higher income level who's not subsidy eligible trying to buy her own policy. We should definitely be looking at the way that you described it, that global number of what percentage of people's income are they spending to get their health insurance coverage and to pay for their out-of-pocket costs for their healthcare and consider what's affordable and recognize that people at the lower end don't have the ability to pay as high a percentage of their income toward that care and that coverage as people with a higher income.

Senator CASSIDY. Mr. Hudak, you have a comment?

Mr. HUDAK. Yes. I want to just point out as part of our business of advising small businesses, as an accountant, more than 10 years ago, we probably did a financial analysis on HSAs hundreds and hundreds of times, and the way it worked is when you buy an HSA compliant plan, it provided no first dollar benefits except for the exception of prevention. Because of that, the way the HSA was cost, the savings in premiums would allow those contributions by the employer into an HSA account on behalf of the employee to give them the flexibility to use those dollars.

Today, that's impossible to do. An employer not only has to deal with the insanity of the premium increases, but they don't have the ability to assist the employees in that way again, because the Affordable Care Act says—mandates that an HSA plan must provide those first dollar benefits. It's priced where an HSA no longer makes any sense. Some can argue that some of these plans—none of them make any sense from a financial perspective except for people who are running away from the tax penalty for not having a compliant plan. That's unbelievable to me.

Senator ENZI. Mr. Glause, did you want to comment?

Mr. GLAUSE. Thank you, Chairman, yes. The deductibles for ACA plans are, in my opinion, extremely high—$6,350. The average person in Wyoming only spends $7,000 on healthcare annually, almost equal to the cost of the deductible. In many cases, these high deductibles are directly related to uncompensated care. Individuals just do not have the money to afford that deductible. Our healthcare facilities are then having to absorb that cost, and in many cases, it's raising the cost of healthcare.

The providers are pretty sure that they're not going to get that first $6,000. They're building that into their rates, and it's caused the rates of healthcare to go up and uncompensated care to go up, which is threatening the existence of the sparse healthcare facilities that we do have in Wyoming.

Senator ENZI. When we were first discussing healthcare changes, there were 49 million people that were uninsured. Today there are still approximately 30 million people uninsured. It's a different group of uninsured people. The ones that couldn't get insurance before have insurance, and the ones that had insurance can't afford the insurance.

One of the things that comes up in the discussion is the effect of changing the bandwidths. Have any of you noticed an impact from that or have any suggestions for solving that?

Mr. Harte.

Mr. HARTE. I didn't integrate a lot of my comments with regard to age bands, but for the edification of the committee, I will say that ACA declares that a three-to-one ratio is appropriate for small businesses across the United States. Most people would first ask me, "Well, what does that really mean?"

What you can't see right now is what the rate grids look like. The rate grids that are handed to a small employer start off with the age of 21 and go up through the age of 65, and every individual on the health insurance plan follows by that grid. That individual who is 21 versus the one who is age 65. It's a multiple of three or a 300 percent differential.

The majority of healthcare is consumed by those who are older. Those over the age of 50 consume a lot more healthcare than those individuals who are younger than the age of 50. What we're seeing is the premiums for the younger population—and one of the objectives of healthcare reform was to insure the younger population— their premiums are too high. A five-to-one ratio would give greater flexibility to the insurance companies to make sure that they're collecting enough money for the older population to provide for their care while at the same time trying to provide more affordable options for the younger population.

Senator ENZI. Mr. Glause.

Mr. GLAUSE. Thank you, Senator Enzi. What we've observed in Wyoming is with the—is that me?

Senator ENZI. That's just us giving ourselves permission not to speak on the floor.

[Laughter.]

Mr. GLAUSE. With the three bandwidths in the ACA as compared to the five bandwidths in our highrisk pool, we've actually found that the rates for young males with a five bandwidth in our highrisk pool is actually cheaper than getting coverage on the ACA. I think that that has constricted the bandwidth and has led to increased costs for the younger, healthier population.

Senator ENZI. Ms. Lueck.

Ms. LUECK. The other side of that would be if you changed it, it would obviously increase rates for the older population. Overall, we really want to make sure that there are healthier people of all ages in the risk pool so that we have as well balanced a risk pool as possible. But if you're talking about changing the age rating rules now from what they are, you're definitely going to see rate increases for certain groups of people.

When the rating rules went into place, things changed for people as well. Women used to be rated more than men. That's a big change. There are some people that saw lower rates as a result of the changes and some people that saw higher rates, and I think they're just different groups of people.

Senator ENZI. That's the 30 million I was talking about. Mr. Hudak.

Mr. HUDAK. I'm not an economist, but before the ACA, younger people weren't so interested in healthcare. Raising their prices hasn't made them more interested in healthcare.

I do want to mention one thing. Connecticut some years ago had an exchange. The Chamber of Commerce had a small business exchange. If you were an employer, you could sign up for the exchange, and participating in there were all the different carriers, the insurance companies. The employee could select any company and any plan, and it would be billed as a group plan. It was fully medically underwritten. If you fell outside of the medical underwriting guidelines, you went into the risk pool.

I always felt the best way to fund a risk pool would be based on market share of the insurance companies. If Anthem of Connecticut had a 30 percent market share, they would be responsible for funding 30 percent of the risk pool. This was a system set up by the Chamber of Commerce.

I think it's a viable solution. I think it adds flexibility and choice, transparency, and, most importantly, one size fits all wouldn't have to be mandated. In other words, employees could have their choice of flexibility and the employer could be the true hero and provide the coverage that's needed.

Senator ENZI. Just to followup on that, you were talking about the highrisk pool that the State had before?

Mr. HUDAK. Correct.

Senator ENZI. Could you just go into that a little more? I must have missed part of it or something, but I think it was important. Mr. HUDAK. It was fully underwritten, and if you fell outside the underwriting guidelines and didn't qualify for the plan, you would go into the risk pool, and your plan would be subsidized by the risk pool. Everybody—all comers would get—it really addressed the adverse selectivity issue, because now you're dealing with a group plan where the qualifying event is new employment, marital change. You didn't have to worry about people jumping on and off, or if you lost your coverage for some reason. Right now, if for some reason, someone for whatever reason missed a premium bill, and their coverage lapsed, good luck trying to get it back. It's a very scary situation right now.

Senator ENZI. Thank you. Mr. Glause.

Mr. GLAUSE. Thank you. In response to Ms. Lueck's response, I'd also like to point out that open enrollment without regard to preexisting conditions every year also increases cost to all consumers, whether you're young or old or middle aged. When the individuals elect not to obtain coverage until they have a need for it, costs are driven up, whereas if the bandwidth was wider and those individuals that were healthier had the opportunity to get into the insurance market at less cost, we may be able to get them coverage for when they need it without waiting until they had a condition that necessitated insurance.

Senator ENZI. Ms. Lueck.

Ms. LUECK. I just wanted to mention, since the guaranteed avail ability in the individual market and the open enrollment period issue came up, that it's one of the most important changes that's happened since 2014. One of the most popular changes, frankly, if you ask the public, is the fact that people can get access to coverage in the open enrollment period and that they don't get denied or that they don't pay higher premiums because of the fact that they have a preexisting condition.

That was obviously something that was very concerning before to people who had those conditions, and it wasn't just people that had really expensive conditions that experienced those kind of problems. It was people that had taken antidepressants or had had chronic sinus infections. It was really a lot of us that would have faced barriers in the individual market.

Now, we have a situation where small employers have a little bit of the pressure taken off, right, because they don't have to feel like they have to provide coverage. That used to be the case, right? They used to feel especially responsible to provide coverage because they may have employees that have health challenges and that wouldn't have been able to get coverage in the individual market, and now there's a backstop there, that people can get access to that coverage, and the open enrollment period is just a way of making sure that people can't actually enroll whenever they want to. They have to do it at a defined time.

Senator ENZI. Thank you.

Back to Mr. Hudak, did you ever look into the SHOP exchanges? Mr. HUDAK. We did, and it appeared that the plans weren't very price competitive. Selections weren't very abundant, and in our area, my wife would have had to change her doctors, and she's had a preexisting condition for more than 15 years. We've always struggled with keeping coverage, but we've always maintained coverage.

It's always been expensive. But I will say today our monthly costs are far above anything that we've ever faced in the past.

To answer your question about the SHOP exchange, I think the selections aren't there, the choices aren't there, and the networks are limited.

Senator ENZI. Anyone else want to comment on that?

Mr. HARTE. I would say to you, Senator Enzi, that I mentioned earlier that we represent 300 companies throughout New England, and it may be helpful to know that only two of our clients are involved in the SHOP. When I testified before you last year, I shared with you some significant challenges that the SHOP has had. I will share with you today that under the leadership of Mr. Counihan, the SHOP is better today than it was a year ago.

However, it still presents the challenges outlined by Mr. Hudak, that sometimes you're going to find within certain States lack of options. You will find bifurcated networks, and sometimes you just don't find the solutions. It does attract a certain employer with less than 25 lives and an average income of less than $50,000 so you can take advantage of tax credits. But the ultimate question for a small business owner like Mr. Hudak will be: Is the aggravation going to be worth it?

Senator ENZI. Thank you. Ms. Lueck.

Ms. LUECK. I just wanted to say something, because I happen to agree with a lot of the panelists—I thought I would take my chance while I could—that the SHOP has obviously experienced a lot of challenges across the country in terms of getting started on time and working well. It had a lot of technical and operational problems when it first started. The reports that I've heard since, in the last year, are that it's better, and that a lot of those problems are resolved. But, of course, the enrollment still remains quite low.

Small employers still have a lot of different options. They can keep buying coverage as they always have done on the open market directly from insurers through their brokers. That's still an option, and they don't have to go to the SHOP. It remains to be seen whether enrollment picks up there, whether there are more concerted efforts to educate employers, or to continue to bring more brokers into the SHOP marketplace, because that's another area where things have gotten better, but perhaps the brokers could have a larger role in the SHOP and that would help get more employers enrolled.

The verdict is still out on the SHOP, and we'll have to wait and see what happens. Clearly, the enrollment has skewed toward those that are eligible for the tax credit that you can get when you're in the SHOP. If we want to assist the very small employers that are eligible a little bit more, maybe that's something to consider.

Senator ENZI. Thank you. Mr. Glause.

Mr. GLAUSE. I'd just like to reiterate what I said in my opening comments, that in Wyoming, we have less than 300 lives covered in the SHOP, and the employers are telling us it's difficult to determine what the tax benefits are. It's convoluted, and they just aren't able to figure out what advantage, if any, there is to providing coverage under the SHOP. At least in our small State, we just haven't seen the benefits to date of the SHOP program.

Ms. LUECK. Just one benefit I'll mention, for what it's worth. There is the ability in the SHOP to offer a defined contribution toward coverage. There's the ability to compare different plans. Obviously, the options are variable, depending upon the market and the State that you're in and the number of carriers that you have access to. But a number of SHOPs do have access to—they present access to multiple carriers so that small businesses can choose from those.

They also have the advantage of not requiring, at least in the federally run shop, a contribution requirement from the small business. So often, we hear this idea that, oh, small businesses just want to provide a little assistance with the premium cost or to help their employees a little bit with the cost. That's an option in the SHOP, and those were the kinds of things that the SHOP was created for, and then, of course, the option to do employee choice and let employees choose either different plans in the same level or among different carriers on their own without the employer making those choices for them. That's a huge change and a new benefit, es pecially for small employers who haven't been able to do that in the past.

Senator ENZI. Mr. Hudak.

Mr. HUDAK. I do want to mention that being able to provide healthcare in a flexible way is very important to small businesses. The No. 1 issue is, right now, one in three businesses have a position open that they can't fill. Trying to attract and retain key people is critical to our success. Great businesses are built with great people. We need to see flexibility in the healthcare system so that we can be inventive. We are finding that younger people like choices, like to be able to spend money—allow them to be true consumers.

We hear this time and time again, and when the little guy is up against the big guy, it's very difficult for us to compete, and the only way we can compete with the limited dollars we have is with flexibility. That's why we believe HRAs are really critical to this puzzle. HRAs allow us to have the flexibility to let them purchase premiums, insurance plans, and a whole host of other benefits. But they are in the driver's seat, and there's a perceived and real value to being in the driver's seat when it comes to your healthcare.

Senator ENZI. Ms. Lueck, in your opening comments, you mentioned the need for transparency of cost. Mr. Harte mentioned that in New Hampshire, they have transparency of cost. Does anybody know if that's available in any other States that way?

I know of a couple of companies that testified before us before that were big enough that they could do those kinds of comparisons within their company. But I'd like to know more about this transparency.

Mr. Harte, you talked about that app.

Mr. HARTE. In answer to your question, do other States have transparency tools, I want to answer that question, definitively, yes. However, I thought it might be helpful to also help you understand how New Hampshire was a bit of a pioneer in healthcare cost transparency, because approximately 10 to 13 years ago, the State of New Hampshire Insurance Department under the leadership of Roger Sevigny came up with *www.nhhealthcost.org*, and it was a limited healthcare cost transparency tool.

The first thing I'll share with you, Mr. Chairman, is that the first step could be that some of the States, through the insurance departments, can learn from the model in the State of New Hampshire, whereby the transparency conversation can start. That being said, the insurance industry is embracing the concept of helping their health plan members to have access to this information. As I shared with you before, the differentials can be greater than 600 percent from one facility to another, and, quite frankly, the lower cost facility can possibly be the higher quality of the two.

There are some significant large companies who are in this mar ketplace right now, which I will share with you after today's hearing. But, also, health plans across the country are starting to get into the business of healthcare cost transparency.

Senator ENZI. Mr. Glause.

Mr. GLAUSE. I was just going to echo Mr. Harte's comments. There are a number of States that have created either an allclaims database or a multiclaims—multipayers claims database. The problem is that research has not borne out that these allpayer claims databases or multipayer claims databases have reduced cost. Even in certain instances, in California, we've seen them increase cost.

I think the real challenge with the allpayer claims database is figuring out how to incentivize that for individuals. For instance, there is a Neiman Marcus approach to it, that if someone charges more, they must be better. It has to have a quality concept tied to it. And, as well, the individuals who have fulfilled their deductible—they no longer have any skin in the game. We have to figure out how to incentivize it.

The other issue it creates is the providers have access to it as well, and you sometimes see providers bringing up their cost to meet the higher cost rather than bringing them down in limited competition areas.

Senator ENZI. Thank you.

I'll have some other questions that are probably a lot more specific, and so I'll submit those.

[The information referred to follows:] [SUBCOMMITTEE INSERT]

Senator ENZI. But does anybody want to make a closing comment?

Mr. Harte.

Mr. HARTE. Thank you, Senator Enzi. Again, thank you for having me here today. I don't want this hearing to end without me talking about a couple of issues that are of great concern to my employer clients, one of which is the employer mandate and the management and administration of the employer mandate. Many employers issued their first tax forms just a few months ago, and the burden on employers from 50 and up is overwhelming at best.

The volume of hours, administration, and management for any employer, regardless of size, to administer the employer mandate is overwhelming. Many employers, large employers, went to their payroll company last July and said, "I need to start preparing for the employer mandate and my reporting. Can you help me with that?" Now, as we know, a lot of healthcare reform reporting requires that hours be submitted on a monthly basis for individual employees. The clearinghouse for that is a payroll company.

Many payroll companies shut down their clients and said, "I apologize. We cannot do your employer reporting," which left thousands of employers across this country looking for a third party solution without access to all that data, and they didn't talk to each other. My hope is that in this coming year, there will be better solutions so that the employers are not so overwhelmed.

My other comment to you, Senator Enzi, is I wanted to share some concern that I have with regard to the consideration of eliminating the employer exclusion. As many of us know, the employer exclusion says that if a small business, like Mr. Hudak, contributes premiums toward their employees' health insurance benefits, then that benefit, the dollar benefit of the health insurance plan, is excluded from an individual's income.

I will share with you, anecdotally, some of my clients. One of my clients is a large State employees union, and all of their employees will be subject to a significant tax increase absent the employer exclusion. In addition, as we're here today talking more about small businesses, since the rate grids came out, we have seen some significant discrimination in local businesses, because they look at these rate grids, and they say, "It costs more to hire someone and provide benefits to someone who is age 55 and older."

What you'll also find by eliminating the employer exclusion is that there will be further discrimination amongst people who are my age and older, because when you work for a small business, if the volume of premium paid for that individual is higher than others, then, conversely, the tax to the business, for the payroll tax, as well as the individual tax to the employee, will be significant.

I actually have some examples here that one taxable income for a 25 yearold will be an additional $12,900—and this is a reallife example from one of my clients—versus a $29,000 additional income, almost like imputed income. Take their Federal tax rate of anywhere from 10 percent to 39.6 percent, and you're going to have a substantial tax burden to individuals.

My concern, Senator Enzi, as you've known me through the years, my platform is we need to make health insurance more affordable. If in the event that we eliminate the employer exclusion, we will absolutely see an increase in the number of uninsured, because it will be significantly more unaffordable than you have it today. You'll also have employers who say, like Senator Scott said earlier, why don't employers just pay the $2,000 penalty?

In my conversations with my clients every year, when I sit down and share with them a 10 percent to 30 percent increase, they're already considering walking away from their health insurance plan. By eliminating the employer exclusion, I can assure you that we will see a massive exodus from the small employer marketplace and the large employer marketplace by employers who are desperately concerned about the impact of losing the employer exclusion.

Senator ENZI. Thank you.

I appreciate all the comments today and all of the suggestions. I've got five pages of things circled here to followup on and see if we can work them into, again, making things more affordable for people that work for small businesses, because that's what we're trying to do, and I know a lot of people want to do that.

I want to thank you all for your testimony and the ideas and suggestions. I hope I got them right. But they're very good. You're a knowledgeable group, and perhaps we'll have some more questions submitted for you. They have to be given to my office by close of business on Tuesday, July 5, 2016.

Thank you very much. The roundtable is adjourned.

[Additional material follows.]

Additional Material Prepared Statement of Senator Hatch

Small businesses in Utah, and across our Nation, are an important source of employment and economic activity while serving as the foundation of our communities. According to the Small Business Administration, Utah small businesses employ more than 520,000 individuals, which is nearly half of the private sector workforce. Firms with fewer than 100 employees make up the largest share of small businesses in Utah. Small businesses spark innovation, create jobs and complement the economic activity of large organizations. However, small business creation and growth is faltering in Utah and throughout the country because of the Affordable Care Act and its increased costs.

According to a study conducted by the National Federation of Independent Business Research Foundation, "the cost of health insurance is the most critical concern for small business owners in operating their business . . ." This is further exacerbated by mandates and taxes imposed by Obamacare. It is time for the Federal Government to stop this assault on small businesses and hardworking Americans. Through my work as a member of this committee, as Chairman of the Finance Committee, and as a Utahn seeking common sense solutions to unnecessarily complex prob lems, I have fought to decrease health care costs for small businesses in a variety of ways.

At the end of 2015, I ensured that Obamacare's 40 percent excise tax on high cost employer-sponsored health benefits—referred to as the Cadillac Tax—was delayed until 2020. Similarly, I worked to enact a 1 year moratorium on the health insurance tax, which is estimated to increase premiums on average for small employers by more than $200 per employee. While these are small steps to address the rising cost of health care, they provided meaningful relief in the short term.

As Chairman of the Finance Committee, I have also worked with my colleague, Senator Chuck Grassley, to support the Small Business Health Care Relief Act (S. 3060). This measure would allow small businesses that have no more than 50 employees to offer standalone Health Reimbursement Accounts (HRAs) to their employees if certain conditions are met without subjecting them to an onerous excise tax that went into effect last July. HRAs are an important tool used by employers to help employees pay for health insurance premiums and medical expenses. I will continue to work with Senator Grassley on avenues to advance this important piece of legislation.

Many of the other ideas I believe will help to decrease health care costs for small businesses are included in the Patient Choice, Affordability, Responsibility, and Empowerment (CARE) Act I proposed with my colleagues, Senator Richard Burr and Congressman Fred Upton. The

Patient CARE Act would repeal Obamacare, and instead build the economy, empower the individual, and reduce health care costs. Of particular interest for employers should be the repeal of the employer mandate that imposes a onesize fits all requirement on small businesses that offer health insurance coverage to their employees. Small businesses know their employees and their health needs better than Federal bureaucrats in Washington, and should have flexibility to design benefit packages that work best for them. Furthermore, this proposal would allow small businesses to join together to negotiate small business health plans to leverage purchasing power, which could help expand access to coverage and lower health care costs.

Another component of the Patient CARE Act is giving employers and employees more access to Consumer Directed Health Plans, also known as HSAEligible Health Plans. As the lead sponsor of the Health Savings Act of 2016, I feel strongly that giving employees more choice and greater control of their earnings will enable smarter, more personal decisions about their health needs.

Starting, maintaining and growing a small business demands hard work, dedication, and focus. The Federal Government should do all it can to support small business employers and employees, rather than increasing burdensome regulations that make it difficult for businesses to grow and hire more workers. I will continue to advocate for ways to bend the cost curve for small businesses purchasing health insurance coverage, and I invite anyone—Republican or Democrat—to work with me to address rising health care costs, which is a top issue facing the economic engines of our country.

[Whereupon, at 3:25 p.m., the hearing was adjourned.]

In: Health Care Costs for Consumers … ISBN: 978-1-53616-862-4
Editor: Maik Nacht

Chapter 3

BUREAU OF PRISONS: BETTER PLANNING AND EVALUATION NEEDED TO UNDERSTAND AND CONTROL RISING INMATE HEALTH CARE COSTS*

United States Government Accountability Office

WHY GAO DID THIS STUDY

As of June 2017, BOP was responsible for the custody and care—including health care—of about 154,000 inmates housed in BOP institutions. Health care includes medical, dental, and psychological treatment. BOP provides most care inside its institutions, but transports inmates outside when circumstances warrant. GAO was asked to review health care costs at BOP institutions.

* This is an edited, reformatted and augmented version of United States Government Accountability Office; Report to Congressional Requesters, Publication No. GAO-17-379, dated June 2017.

This report addresses: (1) BOP's costs to provide health care services and factors that affect costs; (2) the extent to which BOP has data to help control health care costs; and (3) the extent to which BOP has planned and implemented cost control efforts.

GAO analyzed BOP health care obligations data for fiscal years 2009 through 2016, gathered information on BOP's health care cost control initiatives through a data collection instrument, and reviewed BOP's health care related strategic plans. GAO also interviewed BOP officials and visited 10 BOP institutions, selected in part, for total and per capita medical services costs.

What GAO Recommends

GAO is making five recommendations, including that BOP conduct a cost- effectiveness analysis to identify the most effective method to collect health care utilization data; conduct a spend analysis of health care spending data; evaluate cost control initiatives; and enhance its planning efforts by incorporating elements of a sound planning approach. BOP concurred with the recommendations.

What GAO Found

From fiscal years 2009 through 2016, the Bureau of Prisons (BOP) obligated more than $9 billion for the provision of inmate health care and several factors affected these costs. Obligations for health care rose from $978 million in fiscal year 2009 to $1.34 billion in fiscal year 2016, an increase of about 37 percent. On a per capita basis, and adjusting for inflation, health care obligations rose from $6,334 in fiscal year 2009 to $8,602 in fiscal year 2016, an increase of about 36 percent. BOP cited an aging inmate population, rising pharmaceutical prices, and increasing costs of outside medical services as factors that accounted for its overall costs.

Bureau of Prisons (BOP) institution obligations for inmate health care, including psychological care, and inflation adjusted per capita obligations from fiscal years 2009 through 2016

	Fiscal year							
	2009	2010	2011	2012	2013	2014	2015	2016
Total health care obligations (millions)	$978	$1,035	$1,081	$1,122	$1,200	$1,243	$1,299	$1,344
Per capita obligations (2016 dollars)	$6,334	$6,495	$6,485	$6,627	$6,998	$7,350	$7,958	$8,602

Source: GAO analysis of BOP data. | GAO-17-379.

BOP lacks or does not analyze certain health care data necessary to understand and control its costs. For example, while BOP's data can show how much BOP is spending overall on health care provided inside and outside an institution, BOP lacks utilization data, which is data that shows how much it is spending on individual inmate's health care or how much it is expending on a particular health care service. BOP has identified potential solutions for gathering utilization data, but has not conducted a cost-effectiveness analysis of these solutions to identify the most effective solution. BOP also does not analyze health care spending data, i.e., what its institutions are buying, from whom, and how much they spend. BOP has pursued some opportunities to control its health care spending through interagency collaboration and national contracts, but it has not conducted a spend analysis to better understand trends. Doing so would provide BOP with better information to acquire goods and services more strategically.

BOP has initiatives aimed to control health care costs but could better assess effectiveness and apply a sound planning approach. Since 2009, BOP has implemented or planned a number of initiatives related to health care cost control, but has not evaluated their cost-effectiveness. Further, BOP has engaged in a strategic planning process to help control costs, but has not incorporated certain elements of a sound planning approach, such as developing a means to measure progress toward its objectives and identifying the resources and investments needed for its initiatives. By incorporating these elements, BOP could enhance its planning and implementation efforts before expending resources, better positioning itself for success as it aims to control health care costs.

ABBREVIATIONS

AASLD	American Association for the Study of Liver Diseases
BEMR	Bureau Electronic Medical Record
BOP	Bureau of Prisons
BOPMOP	BOP Mail Order Pharmacy
CT	Computerized tomography
DOJ	Department of Justice
FCC	Federal Correctional Complex
FCI	Federal Correctional Institution
FDA	Food and Drug Administration
FDC	Federal Detention Center
FMC	Federal Medical Center
FMIS	Financial Management Information System
FPDS-NG	Federal Procurement Data System-Next Generation
FSS	Federal Supply Schedule
FTC	Federal Transfer Center
HIV/AIDS	Human immunodeficiency virus/acquired immunodeficiency syndrome
HSD	Health Services Division
JMD	Justice Management Division
MCC	Metropolitan Correctional Center
MCFP	Medical Center for Federal Prisoners
MRI	Magnetic resonance imaging
NHE	National health expenditures
NHEA	National Health Expenditure Accounts
OIG	Office of Inspector General
OMB	Office of Management and Budget
RDAP	Residential Drug Abuse Program
SOC	Sub-Object Classification

USP	U.S. Penitentiary
VA	Department of Veterans Affairs

June 29, 2017

The Honorable Charles E. Grassley
Chairman
Committee on the Judiciary
United States Senate

The Honorable Claire McCaskill
Ranking Member
Committee on Homeland Security and Governmental Affairs
United States Senate

The mission of the Department of Justice's (DOJ) Federal Bureau of Prisons (BOP) is to protect society by confining offenders in facilities that are safe, humane, cost-efficient, and appropriately secure. As part of its duties, BOP is responsible for delivering adequate health care, including medical, dental, and mental health care, in a manner consistent with accepted community standards for a correctional environment.[1] BOP reported obligating almost $1.2 billion of its $6.9 billion appropriation to the medical and dental care of inmates for fiscal year 2016.[2] These costs include various categories, such as medical, dental, and psychiatric staff salaries within BOP institutions; pharmaceuticals and medical supplies; and expenses associated with inmates receiving care at a local health care

[1] BOP's Health Services Administration Program Statement states that BOP is to deliver medically necessary health care to inmates in accordance with proven standards of care. See BOP Program Statement 6010.05, *Health Services Administration*, June 26, 2014.

[2] An obligation is a definite commitment that creates a legal liability of the government for the payment of goods and services received. BOP combines medical, dental, and psychiatric care in its reporting of medical services obligations. Mental health care is reported separately in its Psychology Services obligations. The $6.9 billion appropriation is for the Salaries and Expenses portion of BOP's fiscal year 2016 annual appropriation and does not include the separate Buildings and Facilities appropriation for fiscal year 2016.

provider, such as a hospital, when BOP cannot provide the necessary care in-house.[3] In addition, for fiscal year 2016, BOP reported obligating more than $70 million to provide mental health treatment to inmates, including psychological treatment such as group and individual psychotherapy sessions, psychology treatment programs, and sex offender treatment programs.[4] BOP's fiscal year 2017 Congressional Budget Justification shows medical services and psychological services funding increasing annually, and BOP expects costs to continue to increase in the future, driven by, among other things, rising costs across the health care industry, including pharmaceutical costs, and the expanded needs of the aging inmate population.

Multiple U.S. courts over the years have determined that inmates have a constitutional right to adequate medical and mental health care.[5] By statute, BOP is required to provide for suitable housing and the safekeeping, care, and subsistence of all persons charged with or convicted of offenses against the United States.[6] In light of the importance of providing health care to BOP inmates, and the rising costs associated with providing care, you asked us for information on BOP's costs for inmate health care, factors that are impacting costs, and what initiatives BOP has undertaken to address rising costs. This report addresses the following questions: (1) How much did BOP obligate for inmate health care from fiscal years 2009 through 2016 and what factors affect BOP's costs? (2) To what extent does BOP have data available to understand and help control its health care costs? (3) What initiatives has BOP identified and

---

[3] BOP distinguishes between medical services and psychology services, which are accounted for separately in BOP's budget. Psychiatric staff salaries are included in medical services obligations as psychiatrists have the authority to prescribe medication.

[4] See our prior work on BOP inmate mental health care. GAO, *Bureau of Prisons: Timelier Reviews, Plans for Evaluations, and Updated Policies Could Improve Inmate Mental Health Services Oversight*, GAO-13-1 (Washington, D.C.: July 17, 2013).

[5] For example, the United States Supreme Court held in the case of *Brown v. Plata,* 563 U.S. 493, 497 (2011), that adequate medical and mental health care must meet minimum constitutional requirements and meet prisoners' basic health needs. Similarly, the United States Supreme Court concluded in the case of *Estelle v. Gamble*, 429 U.S. 97, 104 (1976), that deliberate indifference to the serious medical needs of prisoners by prison personnel constitutes the unnecessary and wanton infliction of pain prohibited by the Eighth Amendment.

[6] 18 U.S.C. § 4042(a)(2).

implemented to help control health care costs and how effectively has BOP planned its health care cost control efforts?

To address these questions, we interviewed BOP officials knowledgeable about health care costs and cost control efforts from several divisions and offices, as well as officials at BOP's six regional offices. We conducted site visits to 10 BOP institutions, and selected these institutions based, in part, on factors that both BOP and existing research indicated could be affecting costs, such as inmate characteristics and geography, as well as other factors that allowed for variation in our sample (see app. I for more details on our selection criteria). In addition, we reviewed key documents, such as BOP's Congressional Budget Justifications for fiscal years 2009 through 2018.

To examine how much BOP has obligated for inmate health services over the past 8 fiscal years and the factors that affect BOP's costs, we reviewed key documents, such as BOP's Annual Financial Statements, and the Department of Justice's Financial Management Information System Sub-Object Classification (SOC) Code Guide.[7] We also analyzed BOP obligation data from fiscal years 2009 through 2016 on medical services, psychology services, drug and sex offender treatment programs, and medical staff training. We included 8 years of obligations data in order to observe trends over time in health care costs. We included all categories of care that are considered essential to treating health, including mental health and substance use disorder treatment. To determine the per capita obligations, we divided the total obligation by the inmate population at the end of each fiscal year. We adjusted these data to reflect health care inflation. To better understand the composition of medical services obligations, we analyzed obligations by SOC code. To understand the changes in pharmaceutical expenditures over the period we reviewed, as well as what illnesses were impacting those obligations, we analyzed BOP's list of top 50 medications for fiscal years 2009 through 2016. We compared these medications to the U.S. National Library of Medicine's

---

[7] Federal agencies use SOC Code Guides to standardize budgetary information. SOC codes define the nature of services or articles obligated, and include codes for items such as personnel compensation, rent, supplies, and contractual services.

MedlinePlus list of drugs and supplements, in order to determine their uses.[8] To assess the reliability of BOP's obligations and expenditures data, we performed electronic testing for obvious errors in accuracy and completeness, and interviewed agency officials knowledgeable about BOP's budget to determine the processes in place to ensure the integrity of the data. We determined that the data were sufficiently reliable for the purposes of this report. Finally, since geographic location may impact the provision or cost of inmate health care, we analyzed BOP institutions' proximity to hospitals.[9] To do this, we used geographic information services software to map the addresses of all BOP institutions, and identify how many hospitals were within a 20 mile radius of the institution.

To examine the extent to which BOP has data available to understand and help control its health care costs, the initiatives BOP has identified and implemented to help control health care costs, and how effectively BOP has planned and implemented these initiatives, we reviewed relevant BOP program statements. We also conducted interviews with BOP officials knowledgeable about cost control initiatives. Further, we reviewed Office of Management and Budget (OMB) guidance on cost- effectiveness analysis and BOP policies to assess the extent to which BOP analyzed its efforts to gather data. To determine the extent of available data on BOP health care spending, we searched the Federal Procurement Data System-Next Generation (FPDS-NG) for BOP contract actions for fiscal years 2009 through 2015 and obtained pharmaceutical obligations data from BOP for that same period.[10] Based on these steps, we determined the data were sufficiently reliable for the purposes of our reporting objective.

---

[8] MedlinePlus, produced by the National Library of Medicine, is the National Institutes of Health's website that contains extensive information on prescription and nonprescription drugs, in addition to information on over 1,000 diseases and conditions.

[9] For the purposes of our analysis, a hospital is defined as a building or building complex providing general medical or surgical inpatient care. It includes general hospitals, specialty hospitals (such as cancer, maternity, substance abuse, psychiatric, and rehabilitation hospitals). It does not include psychiatric or behavioral facilities that are not hospitals, long-term care medical centers or nursing homes, walk-in centers or outpatient clinics, imaging centers, medical doctors' offices, and rehabilitation centers.

[10] FPDS-NG is a single source for U.S. government-wide procurement data. Managed by the General Services Administration, it is the central repository of information on federal contracting. The system contains detailed information on contract actions over $3,500.

To determine how well BOP's health care cost control planning mechanisms work, we obtained and reviewed selected portions of the annual BOP-wide strategic plans for 2009 through 2015, BOP's Health Services Division (HSD) Governing Board Meeting Minutes through 2015, and the HSD Strategic Plan for 2015 through 2019. To identify BOP's health care cost control efforts, their status of implementation, and the extent to which BOP had conducted cost estimates for each, we interviewed BOP officials and reviewed documents they provided, as well as reviewed relevant GAO reports and DOJ Office of Inspector General (OIG) reports.[11] We summarized this information into a data collection instrument for verification by BOP officials and requested additional data and supporting documentation for each initiative. We also interviewed officials from DOJ OIG and DOJ's Justice Management Division[12] to discuss prior DOJ report recommendations on BOP health care costs. We interviewed officials at the 10 institutions we visited, observed health care programs and cost control efforts, and obtained documents relating to the costs and cost savings of regional and institutional initiatives to control health care costs. Appendix I contains a more detailed discussion of our objectives, scope, and methodology.

We conducted this performance audit from February 2016 to June 2017 in accordance with generally accepted government auditing standards. Those standards require that we plan and perform the audit to obtain sufficient, appropriate evidence to provide a reasonable basis for our findings and conclusions based on our audit objectives. We believe that the evidence obtained provides a reasonable basis for our findings and conclusions based on our audit objectives.

---

[11] See for example: GAO, *Bureau of Prisons: Information on Efforts and Potential Options to Save Costs*, GAO-14-821 (Washington, D.C.: Sept. 30, 2014). DOJ OIG, *The Federal Bureau of Prison's Efforts to Manage Inmate Health Care*, Audit Report 08-08 (Washington, D.C.: Feb. 2008); and *Follow-Up Audit of the Federal Bureau of Prisons' Efforts to Manage Inmate Health Care*, Audit Report 10-30 (Washington, D.C.: July 2010).

[12] DOJ's Justice Management Division (JMD) provides DOJ with advice on policy for budget and financial management, program evaluation, auditing, personnel management and training, procurement, information processing and telecommunications, security, and for all matters pertaining to organization, management, and administration. In 2012, JMD budget staff issued an assessment of BOP's method for procuring medical services and potential ways to reduce costs, including cost savings opportunities.

BACKGROUND

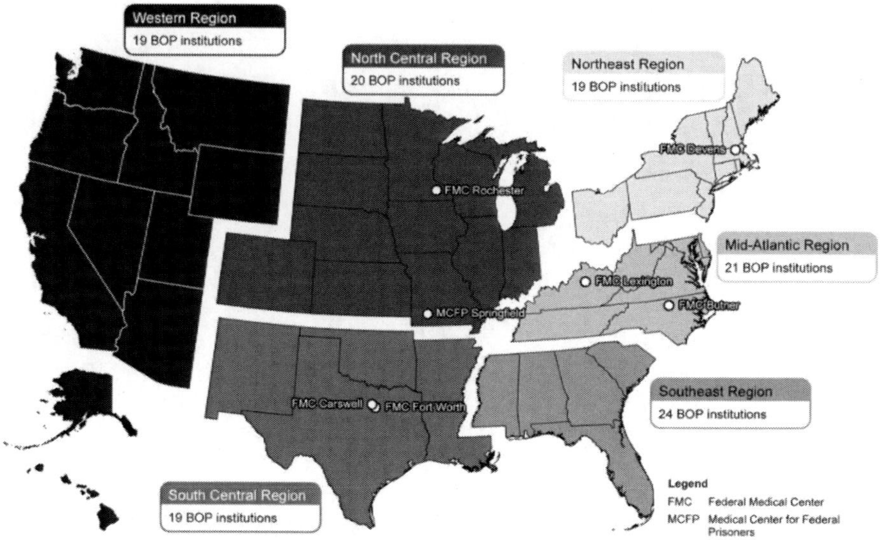

Source: GAO analysis of BOP data; Map Resources (map). | GAO-17-379.

Note: Six of the medical referral centers are named Federal Medical Center (FMC) and one is named United States Medical Center for Federal Prisoners (MCFP). According to BOP, there is no salient difference in the medical mission for the seven institutions and therefore all can be referred to as FMCs.

Figure 1. Bureau of Prisons' (BOP) Regions, Number of Institutions per Region, and Locations of Federal Medical Centers.

As of June 2017, BOP was responsible for approximately 188,000 inmates in federal custody. About 81 percent, or approximately 154,000 inmates, are housed in BOP-operated institutions.[13] There are 122 BOP-operated institutions, with some of the institutions clustered in a Federal

[13] BOP also has inmates in privately run facilities and other types of facilities such as Residential Reentry Centers (RRC). We excluded the privately managed facilities from our review as BOP does not track the specific costs for health care provided to inmates housed therein. Rather, BOP uses fixed-price contracts that only require the contractors to provide BOP with their costs on a per inmate per day basis. We also excluded RRCs from our scope as, according to BOP officials, BOP does not cover health care expenses for all inmates housed in RRCs as some inmates receive care through employer-provided insurance or other means.

Correctional Complex (FCC).[14] BOP designates 7 of its 122 institutions as medical referral centers, generally called a Federal Medical Center (FMC), to provide advanced care for inmates with more serious chronic or acute medical conditions.[15] Each BOP institution (or complex) is located within one of six regions, with an office overseeing the region (see Figure 1). BOP also has a Central Office, located in Washington, D.C., that oversees the six regions.

Provision of Health Care

BOP is responsible for providing medically necessary medical, dental, and mental health services in a manner consistent with standards of care for the non-prison community.[16] BOP's Health Services Division oversees the provision of medical, dental, and psychiatric services. BOP's Psychology Services Branch, under its Reentry Services Division, is responsible for providing psychology services, including psychology treatment programs and drug abuse treatment programs.[17]

BOP provides most medical and dental care inside its institutions (inside care), usually with BOP-employed medical staff. The level and kinds of services provided depends upon the care level of the institution, as described below. Each BOP institution operates a health services unit.

---

[14] At FCCs, institutions with different missions (for example, medical/mental health, pretrial, and holdover) and security levels are located in proximity to one another. FCCs could be made up of two institutions, or up to four institutions. In total, there are 15 complexes.

[15] Six of the medical referral centers are named Federal Medical Center (FMC) and one is named United States Medical Center for Federal Prisoners. According to BOP, there is no salient difference in the medical mission for the seven institutions and therefore all can be referred to as FMCs.

[16] BOP distinguishes between medically necessary acute or emergent care, and medically necessary non-emergent care. Medically necessary acute or emergent care is associated with medical conditions that without care would cause rapid deterioration of health, significant irreversible loss of function, or may be life threatening. Medically necessary non-emergent care is associated with conditions that are not immediately life-threatening but which without care could lead to significant risk of deterioration leading to premature death, reduction in the possibility of repair later without present treatment, and significant pain or discomfort that impacts daily living. See: BOP, *Program Statement: Patient Care*, Number: 6031.04 (June 3, 2014).

[17] See GAO-13-1.

Most units have examination rooms, treatment rooms, dental clinics, radiology and laboratory areas, a pharmacy, and administrative offices, as can be seen in Figure 2 below. BOP staffs these health units with medical professionals including physicians, dentists, nurses, pharmacists, and mid-level practitioners.[18] Inside care services include:

- Health screening upon inmates' admission to the prison, comprehensive documentation of inmates' medical history, and physical exams to identify underlying infectious, chronic, and behavioral health needs.
- Sick call triage and episodic visits to assess, diagnose, and treat short-term health problems.
- Preventative health visits to screen for underlying chronic conditions and immunize against transmission of preventable infectious diseases.
- Chronic care clinics to manage long-term diseases, such as diabetes, asthma, and congestive heart failure.
- Rehabilitative care to regain or maintain optimal physical and mental health function.
- Oral health care to assess, diagnose, treat, and prevent dental cavities and oral diseases.

When BOP is unable to provide a medical service to an inmate, BOP transports the inmate to a medical facility or provider in the community (outside care). Generally, each BOP institution has its own outside care contract that sets payment rates for services provided with the contracted community medical centers and providers. Further, apart from some national BOP contracts that standardize goods and services,[19] each BOP institution acquires its own health care goods and services. Institution-acquired goods and services vary, and include contracted health care

---

[18] BOP also contracts with medical providers to offer clinics and specialty services inside the institutions to complement the primary care offered by BOP staff. See: BOP, *Program Statement: Patient Care*, Number: 6031.04 (June 3, 2014).

[19] According to BOP, examples of national contracts include the purchase of X-ray equipment, pharmaceuticals, and medical/surgical supplies.

professionals, medical imaging services, such as ultrasound and magnetic resonance imaging, medical equipment, and medical waste disposal.[20]

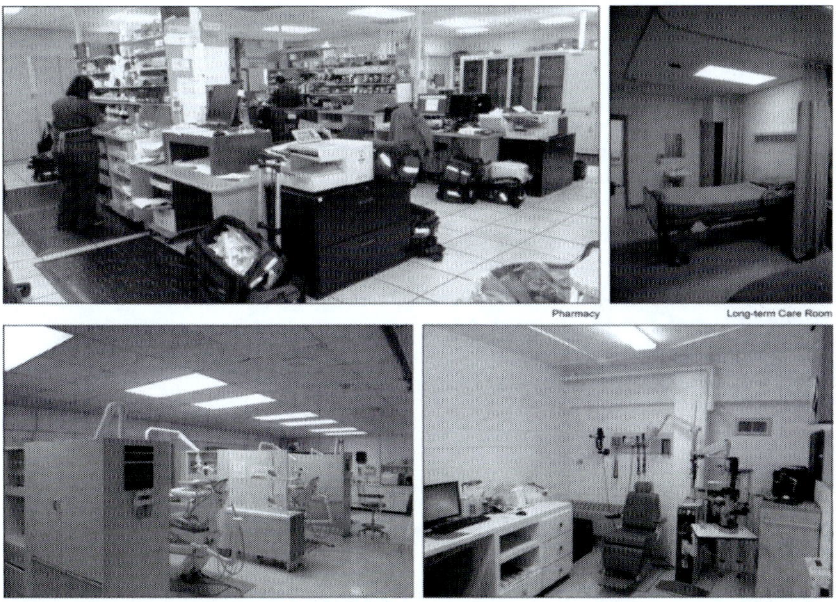

Source: BOP. | GAO-17-379.

Note: These images represent various health care facilities at BOP institutions. They are not necessarily reflective of the facilities at all BOP institutions, which may differ based on medical care level and available resources.

Figure 2. Select Images of Health Services Facilities and Equipment at Bureau of Prisons' (BOP) Institutions.

BOP Institution Care Levels

Beginning the process in 2004, BOP instituted a medical and mental health care level system for its inmates and its institutions. BOP designates inmates as a care level 1, 2, 3, or 4, depending on the level of medical and mental health services required. Inmates designated as a care level 1 are generally considered healthy, and the intensity of care required increases along with care level (see Table 1).

---

[20] BOP relies on contracting for specialty imaging, which could include a computerized tomography (CT) scan or magnetic resonance imaging (MRI). For basic radiographic imaging, over 95 percent of BOP institutions use BOP's teleradiology program.

Table 1. Description of the medical and mental health care levels of Bureau of Prisons' (BOP) inmates

Care level designation	Description	Percentage of inmates at each inmate medical care level (as of March 2017)[a]	Percentage of inmates at each inmate mental care level (as of March 2017)[a]
Care level 1	Medical care level 1 inmates are generally healthy, under 70 years of age, and may have some limited medical needs requiring clinician evaluation and monitoring such as mild asthma or diet-controlled diabetes. Mental care level 1 inmates show no significant level of functional impairment associated with mental illness and demonstrate no need for regular mental health interventions.	69	95
Care level 2	Medical care level 2 inmates are those with stable conditions, requiring at least quarterly clinician evaluation, such as medication-controlled diabetes or emphysema. Mental care level 2 inmates are those requiring routine outpatient mental health care on an ongoing basis and/or need brief, crisis-oriented mental health care of significant intensity.	25	3
Care level 3	Medical care level 3 inmates are fragile outpatients who require frequent clinical contacts, and/or who may require some assistance with activities of daily living. Examples include patients with advanced human immunodeficiency virus/acquired immunodeficiency syndrome (HIV/AIDS) disease or end-stage liver disease. Mental care level 3 inmates are those that require enhanced outpatient mental health care, such as weekly interventions, or placement in a residential Psychology Treatment Program.[b]	2	<1

Care level designation	Description	Percentage of inmates at each inmate medical care level (as of March 2017)[a]	Percentage of inmates at each inmate mental care level (as of March 2017)[a]
Care level 4	Medical care level 4 inmates are severely impaired, and may require daily nursing care, such as patients with cancer in active treatment, dialysis, quadriplegia, and those undergoing or recovering from major surgery. Mental care level 4 inmates are those requiring acute care in a psychiatric hospital.	1	<1

Source: BOP. | GAO-17-379.

[a]Percentage does not equal 100 percent as some inmates were still under an initial care level designation—known as screen level—which is made by BOP's Designation and Sentence Computation Center before arrival at a BOP institution. Upon arrival at a BOP institution, BOP staff determines the care level.

[b]Psychology Treatment Programs typically involve standard protocols that all apply to all participants, including residential and non-residential drug treatment programs, sex offender management programs, and other specialized mental health treatment programs.

BOP also classifies its institutions as a care level 1, 2, 3, or 4, depending on the level of medical and mental health services provided (see app. II for a complete list of institutions with their associated medical care levels). As of 2017, BOP has seven care level 4 institutions—FMCs—that offer advanced care, such as dialysis, oncology treatment, limited surgery services, prosthetics, inpatient and forensic mental health, dementia care, and end-of-life care (see app. III for more information on the FMCs).[21]

BOP Electronic Medical Records System

BOP uses an electronic medical records system—the Bureau Electronic Medical Record (BEMR) system—to keep track of an inmate's medical, social, and psychological history. It includes information on an inmate's clinical encounters (for both inside care and outside care) and

[21] Forensic mental health is the psychological or psychiatric evaluation of pretrial and post- trial inmates pursuant to 18 U.S.C. §§ 4241 – 4247.

medication, among other things.[22] According to BOP officials, BEMR differs from typical electronic medical records systems used outside of prison systems, which generally tie a diagnostic code to a reimbursement rate.[23] BOP's system differs because it was designed as a record of clinical care, not a record of managing reimbursements through private insurance companies, Medicare, or Medicaid.

Health Care Planning and Oversight

BOP plans and oversees its provision of health care through various mechanisms; the following are four major mechanisms that effect health care cost control:

- *HSD Executive Staff:* The HSD Assistant Director, Senior Deputy Assistant Director, and Medical Director oversee the programs, operations, and delivery of health care for BOP institutions. They direct the HSD Branch Chiefs and Chief Professional Officers charged with managing national health programs and services. According to BOP officials, HSD Executive Staff are the most integral planning mechanism and the final decision-makers on any HSD plan.
- *HSD Governing Board:* BOP established this multi-divisional and multi-regional governance structure in 2005 to provide executive level strategic planning and performance evaluation of health services management and operations. Generally, the Board is responsible for overseeing the planning, organization, delivery, and evaluation of health services provided within BOP institutions by BOP staff and contractors. The Board is also tasked with working with HSD to ensure that medically necessary health care is delivered in the most cost-efficient way.

---

[22] An electronic medical records system is defined as an electronic record of health-related information on an individual that can be created, gathered, managed, and consulted by authorized clinicians and staff within one health care organization.

[23] In the United States, every claim submitted by health care providers to health care payers includes International Classification of Diseases (ICD) codes. ICD codes are the standard code set used in the United States documenting medical diagnoses and inpatient procedures.

- *The BOP-Wide Annual Strategic Plan:* BOP develops an annual strategic plan to help fulfill its mission and achieve strategic goals. BOP highlights cost-efficiency in several parts of its annual strategic plan, including its mission and vision statements. BOP's mission statement states that BOP institutions will be cost efficient and BOP's vision statement states that it aims to be the best value provider of efficient correctional services and programs. BOP developed strategic objectives, including a strategic objective focused on health care efficiencies, which BOP explains as "maximizing health care resources as a cost-containment strategy by applying evidence-based business practices and measuring performance through the use of appropriate industry-wide metrics."
- *The HSD Integrated Strategic Plan for 2015 through 2019:* HSD also has an internal five-year strategic plan for the division that focuses on HSD initiatives that are intended to bring large-scale change to BOP's health care system. HSD established four overarching focus areas in the plan: (1) administration and program management, (2) health services staffing and management, (3) financial management, and (4) risk management.[24] The HSD integrated strategic plan includes a description, implementation strategies, and expected outcomes for all four focus areas for each of the 17 HSD branches and sections listed in the plan.

[24] The corresponding goal for each overarching focus area is as follows—(1) Administration and Program Management: To provide effective oversight of Health Services programs, while leveraging the Agency's human capital and technology resources to maximize operational efficiencies and innovate best practices; (2) Health Services Staffing and Management: To build and hire a fully capable and committed workforce by providing meaningful challenges and continuous career development; (3) Financial Management: To effectively manage the Health Services budget through an ongoing analysis of staffing, program efficiencies, and utilization of services to identify opportunities for cost containment presently and in the years ahead; and (4) Risk Management: To identify and mitigate Health Services system vulnerabilities that may jeopardize patient or worker safety.

BOP Obligated More Than $9 Billion for Inmate Health Care from Fiscal Years 2009 through 2016 and Several Factors Affected Costs

BOP's Annual Health Care Obligations Have Increased overall and on a Per Capita Basis

During the 8-year period starting in fiscal year 2009 and ending in fiscal year 2016, BOP obligated more than $9 billion for the provision of inmate health care. According to BOP data, annual obligations increased from a total of almost $978 million in fiscal year 2009 to more than $1.3 billion in fiscal year 2016, an increase of about 37 percent overall during this period (see Table 2). More specifically, annual obligations for medical services[25] increased by about 37 percent, psychology services by about 39 percent, and drug abuse treatment programs by almost 44 percent.[26]

As shown in Table 2, medical services obligations have been increasing over time. Psychology services and drug abuse treatment programs obligations have also been increasing over time. According to BOP officials, more recent increases in psychology services obligations can be attributed to an effort to fill vacancies in psychology services positions throughout BOP institutions. BOP also issued a new program statement in 2014 on the treatment and care of inmates with mental illness, which increased the treatment requirements and necessitated hiring more staff, according to BOP officials.[27] BOP officials also explained that more recent increases in drug abuse treatment program obligations were due to BOP adding 18 additional Residential Drug Abuse Programs (RDAP),

---

[25] Medical services obligations as reported by BOP include medical staff salaries and expenses, medical supplies, pharmaceutical costs, and costs of treating inmates outside of BOP institutions, including overtime costs paid to correctional officers transporting inmates.

[26] Pursuant to 18 U.S.C. § 3621(e), BOP is required to make available appropriate substance abuse treatment for each prisoner the BOP determines has a treatable condition of substance addiction or abuse, including the provision of residential substance abuse treatment for all eligible prisoners (and make arrangements for appropriate aftercare), subject to the availability of appropriations.

[27] BOP, *Program Statement: Treatment and Care of Inmates with Mental Illness*, Number 5310.16 (May 1, 2014).

including some specialized RDAP, beginning in fiscal year 2013. For example, BOP added four RDAPs in high security institutions, and three Spanish- language RDAPs. Sex Offender Management Programs and medical staff training remained fairly constant during this time.

Table 2. Total obligations for inmate health care, population, per capita obligations, and inflation adjusted per capita obligations in Bureau of Prisons (BOP) institutions from fiscal years 2009 through 2016

(Total obligations are in millions of dollars; inmate population and obligations per capita are actual numbers; percentage change is in percent)

Fiscal year	2009	2010	2011	2012	2013	2014	2015	2016
Medical services[a]	$865.2	$914.3	$955.3	$991.0	$1,061.9	$1,096.8	$1,146.7	$1,186.9
Psychology services	$44.7	$47.3	$49.7	$51.6	$52.4	$55.3	$59.4	$62.3
Drug abuse treatment programs	$58.5	$64.1	$66.8	$69.8	$75.9	$79.2	$81.7	$84.0
Sex Offender Management Programs	$6.9	$6.9	$6.6	$7.2	$7.9	$8.7	$9.2	$8.3
Medical staff training	$2.6	$2.5	$2.6	$2.7	$1.8	$3.2	$2.2	$2.7
Total actual health care obligations	$977.9	$1,035.0	$1,081.1	$1,122.3	$1,199.9	$1,243.3	$1,299.2	$1,344.2
Inmate population at end of fiscal year	172,000	172,747	177,368	176,909	176,410	171,868	164,853	156,266
Total annual per capita obligations	$5,686	$5,992	$6,095	$6,344	$6,802	$7,234	$7,881	$8,602
Total annual per capita obligations adjusted for inflation (2016 dollars)	$6,334	$6,495	$6,485	$6,627	$6,998	$7,350	$7,958	$8,602
Percentage change in inflation-adjusted per capita obligations from prior fiscal year	-	2.5	-0.2	2.2	5.6	5.0	8.3	8.1

Source: GAO analysis of BOP data. | GAO-17-379.

Note: Numbers may not total because of rounding.

[a]Medical services obligations as reported by BOP include medical staff salaries and expenses, medical supplies, pharmaceutical costs, and costs of treating inmates outside of BOP institutions, including overtime costs paid to correctional officers transporting inmates.

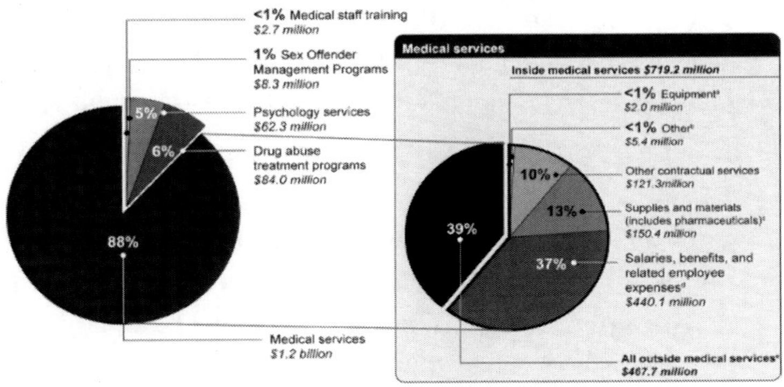

Source: GAO analysis of BOP data. | GAO-17-379.

Note: Numbers may not total because of rounding.

[a]Equipment includes the purchase of personal property of a durable nature. According to BOP officials, under medical services obligations this includes equipment such as X-ray machines, medication dispensing systems, stretchers, telehealth units and peripherals, cardiac monitors/defibrillators, and mini-ambulance carts.

[b]Other includes transportation of items, rent, communications, and utilities, printing and reproduction, grants, subsidies and contributions, and insurance claims.

[c]Supplies and materials include commodities acquired by formal contract or other form of purchase that are ordinarily consumed or expended within one year after they are put to use, converted in the process of construction, or used to form a minor part of equipment. Examples include office supplies, chemicals, surgical and medical supplies, and cleaning supplies. In the case of medical services obligations, the majority of this category is made up of pharmaceuticals.

[d]Salaries, benefits, and related employee expenses include gross compensation for medical staff employed by BOP and the Commissioned Corps Officers of the U.S. Public Health Services (PHS); including paid leave, overtime pay, and holiday pay; benefits such as health and life insurance; and obligations for transportation, per diem, and travel expenses for medical staff while on official duty. PHS is an agency under the Department of Health and Human Services that provides public health services to underserved and vulnerable populations. BOP is responsible for PHS staff working in BOP institutions.

[e]Outside medical services costs include costs to treat inmates at private physicians' offices or at hospitals, as well as transportation costs. These costs include security related costs, including overtime costs for correctional officers to transport the inmates to those locations, as well as for their time guarding inmates, based on inmates' custody levels, when inmates are hospitalized.

Figure 3. Bureau of Prisons' (BOP) Total Health Care Obligations Components, and Total Medical Services Obligations Components for Fiscal Year 2016.

To account for any possible increases in health care obligations as a result of changes in the inmate population,[28] we estimated the annual per capita, or per inmate obligations, by dividing the total health care obligations by the number of inmates—and this figure also increased over time, as can be seen in Table 2. After adjusting for inflation, per capita health care obligations increased from $6,334 per inmate in fiscal year 2009 to $8,602 per inmate in fiscal year 2016, or an increase of about 36 percent during this time period.[29] As Table 2 shows, most of the growth in inflation adjusted per capita obligations occurred in the last four years of fiscal years 2013 through 2016.

Of the five categories we list for total health care obligations (medical services, psychology services, drug treatment programs, Sex Offender Management Programs, and medical staff training) medical services comprised the largest amount, about 88 percent. BOP-reported medical services obligations include several categories of expenditures, which we separated into outside medical services and inside medical services, the latter of which we grouped into five major categories.[30] We analyzed these categories and found that for fiscal year 2016, about 37 percent were for medical staff labor costs inside BOP institutions and 39 percent were for outside medical services, as illustrated in Figure 3. Outside medical services costs include costs to treat inmates at private physicians' offices or at hospitals, as well as transportation costs. These costs include security related costs, including overtime costs for correctional officers to transport the inmates to those locations, as well as for their time guarding inmates, based on inmates' custody levels, when inmates are hospitalized.

---

[28] Between 1980 and 2013, BOP's prison population increased by almost 800 percent. Since 2013, the prison population had begun to decline due to several significant efforts to recalibrate federal sentencing policy, including the retroactive application of revised drug sentencing guidelines, and new charging policies for low-level, non-violent drug offenders. See GAO, *Federal Prison System: Justice Could Better Measure Progress Addressing Incarceration Challenges*, GAO-15-454 (Washington, D.C.: July 19, 2015).

[29] We adjusted the per capita obligations by adjusting every year to 2016 dollars. Before adjusting for inflation, per capita health care obligations increased from $5,686 per inmate in fiscal year 2009 to $8,602 per inmate in fiscal year 2016, or an increase of about 51 percent.

[30] Those categories were: salaries, benefits, and related employee expenses; other contractual services; supplies and materials (which includes pharmaceuticals); equipment; and other.

According to BOP, in fiscal years 2015 and 2016, security related costs made up 19 percent of outside medical services' costs.

At the same time that BOP's health care obligations have been increasing, total United States health care expenditures has also been increasing.[31] According to the Department of Health and Human Services National Health Expenditure Accounts (NHEA) data,[32] total health care expenditures in the United States increased by 5.8 percent in fiscal year 2015, and reached a per capita expenditure of $9,990.[33] However, as we show in Table 3, growth in expenditures, while increasing every year, has not increased consistently, with the last three fiscal years of 2014 through 2016 increasing at a higher rate.[34] Table 3 also shows the per capita expenditures, which have increased every year over the 8-year time period.

---

[31] Expenditures are the actual spending of money. This is different from an obligation, which is a definite commitment that creates a legal liability of the government for the payment of goods and services received.

[32] The U.S. Department of Health and Human Services has published an annual series of data presenting total health expenditures since 1964. The Department completes these estimates with the goal of measuring the total annual dollar amount of health care consumption in the U.S., as well as the dollar amount invested in the medical sector structures and equipment and non-commercial research to procure health services in the future.

[33] National health expenditures (NHE) include, among others, hospital care; physician and clinical services; mental health practitioner services; dental services; other health, residential, and personal care services; home health care; prescription drugs; durable medical equipment; nursing care; and substance abuse facilities. While not directly comparable to health care services in a prison setting, NHE includes most of the same kinds of expenses that are incurred by BOP, such as costs of medical professionals' services and pharmaceuticals.

[34] Higher growth rates in 2014 were primarily due to expansion of private health insurance and Medicaid coverage under the Patient Protection and Affordable Care Act, Pub. L. No. 111-148, 124 Stat. 119 (2010), and to the rapid growth in drug expenditures, including the introduction of new hepatitis C drugs. Higher growth rates in 2015 were due to accelerated growth in spending for private health insurance, hospital care, and physician and clinical services. See: Health Affairs, Anne B. Martin, Micah Hartman, Joseph Benson, Aaron Catlin, and the National Health Expenditure Accounts Team, *National Health Spending in 2014: Faster Growth Driven by Coverage Expansion and Prescription Drug Spending*. Health Affairs published online Dec. 2, 2015, and Anne B. Martin, Micah Hartman, Benjamin Washington, Aaron Catlin, and the National Health Expenditure Accounts Team, *National Health Spending: Faster Growth in 2015 As Coverage Expands And Utilization Increases*. Health Affairs published online Dec. 2, 2016.

Table 3. National health expenditure increases and per capita expenditures from calendar year 2009 through 2016

(Annual growth in percentage and per capita expenditures in actual dollars)								
Calendar year								
	2009	2010	2011	2012	2013	2014	2015	2016[a]
National health expenditures annual percentage growth	4.0	4.1	3.5	4.0	2.9	5.3	5.8	4.8
National health expenditures per capita	$8,141	$8,404	$8,638	$8,915	$9,110	$9,515	$9,990	$10,372

Source: U.S. Department of Health and Human Services. | GAO-17-379.

[a]As of May 2017, national health expenditure figures for 2016 are projections rather than actual figures.

National health expenditures are not directly comparable to BOP's costs because the inmate population is predominantly adult and male, unlike the overall U.S. population. Nevertheless both national health expenditures and BOP health care costs have risen at a higher rate in the last three years.

Various Factors Affected BOP's Health Care Costs

We spoke with numerous BOP officials at the institutional, regional, and Central Office levels to discuss the factors that affected inmate health care costs. Officials frequently cited the following as major factors:

- inmates entering with relatively poorer health,
- aging inmates,
- rising pharmaceutical prices, and
- outside medical services.

Inmates Entering with Relatively Poorer Health

BOP officials stated that inmates are a unique population that poses health care challenges. For example, officials stated that inmates come into the system with more acute needs from limited access to health care or they have engaged in risky behaviors, such as substance abuse. Inmates also tend to have higher rates of infectious diseases and chronic conditions that can persist throughout incarceration. According to the Council of State Governments Justice Center, rates of mental illness, substance use disorders, infectious disease, and chronic health conditions are as much as seven times higher for inmates than rates in the general population.[35]

Aging Inmates

BOP officials stated that an aging inmate population affects health care costs. In a 2015 report, the DOJ OIG also found that aging inmates are more costly to incarcerate than younger inmates due to increased medical needs.[36] BOP data show that the average age of inmates has increased from fiscal year 2009 through 2016, as has the percentage of inmates aged 55 years or older.[37] As seen in Table 4, the percentage of inmates aged 55 years or older increased from 8.4 percent of the population in fiscal year 2009 to 12.0 percent in fiscal year 2016, which is an increase of about 44 percent during this time period.

According to BOP officials, and the 2015 DOJ OIG report, increasing numbers of aging inmates are due to (1) inmates entering the system for the first time at older ages, and (2) inmates aging over time while incarcerated and serving long sentences.[38]

---

[35] Council of State Governments Justice Center, *Medicaid and Financing Health Care for Individuals Involved with the Criminal Justice System*, (New York: Dec. 2013). The Council of State Governments Justice Center is a national nonprofit organization that serves policymakers at the local, state, and federal levels from all branches of government.

[36] DOJ OIG, *The Impact of an Aging Inmate Population on the Federal Bureau of Prisons*, Evaluations and Inspections Division 15-05 (Washington, D.C.: May 2015).

[37] While there is no consensus on what cutoff age is appropriate to be considered an aging inmate, correctional health experts typically define the prison population as "older" at the age of 50 or 55 because inmates generally experience health problems related to aging at a younger age than non-incarcerated people. For the purposes of our report, we are defining "aging inmate" as 55 years of age or older.

[38] DOJ OIG 15-05.

Table 4. Percentage Aged 55 and older, and average age of inmates in Bureau of Prisons (BOP) institutions from fiscal years 2009 through 2016

	Fiscal year							
	2009	2010	2011	2012	2013	2014	2015	2016
Percentage of inmates aged 55 years and older	8.4	8.8	9.3	9.9	10.4	11.0	11.6	12.0
Average inmate age	38.2	38.6	38.9	39.2	39.6	39.9	40.3	40.5

Source: GAO analysis of BOP data. | GAO-17-379.

Note: Fiscal years 2009 through 2015 is GAO analysis of BOP provided data but fiscal year 2016 is BOP-generated data.

Rising Pharmaceutical Prices

Table 5. Bureau of Prisons' (BOP) Pharmaceutical Expenditures Adjusted for Population and Inflation from Fiscal Years 2009 through 2016

(Expenditures are in millions of dollars, per capita expenditures are in actual dollars, and percentage change is in percent)								
	Fiscal year							
	2009	2010	2011	2012	2013	2014	2015	2016
Total pharmaceutical expenditures	$61.4	$64.2	$67.0	$74.1	$79.5	$89.9	$102.3	$111.7
Inmate population at end of the fiscal year	172,000	172,747	177,368	176,909	176,410	171,868	164,853	156,266
Per capita real pharmaceutical expenditures	$357	$371	$378	$419	$451	$523	$621	$715
Per capita pharmaceutical expenditures adjusted for inflation (in 2016 $)	$443	$445	$437	$469	$499	$566	$647	$715
Percentage change in inflation-adjusted per capita pharmaceutical expenditures	-	0.4	-1.7	7.3	6.4	13.4	14.4	10.4

Source: GAO analysis of BOP data. | GAO-17-379.

According to BOP officials, and data we reviewed, expenditures for pharmaceuticals have risen from fiscal years 2009 through 2016. As Table 5 shows, BOP's total pharmaceutical expenditures have increased from $61.4 million in fiscal year 2009 to $111.7 million in fiscal year 2016, or an increase of about 82 percent. Accounting for changes in inmate population over this time period, we found that per capita expenditures have also increased, even in years when population fell. Adjusting for inflation, and using 2016 dollars, we found that overall per capita expenditures increased from $443 per inmate in fiscal year 2009 to $715 in fiscal year 2016, or an increase of about 61 percent.[39]

According to BOP officials, new advances in certain medications—in particular hepatitis C medication, HIV/AIDS medication, and biologics to treat cancers—have contributed to this increase.[40] For example, the Food and Drug Administration (FDA) approved two new medications in a new class of hepatitis C drugs in May 2011, which significantly increased the cost of treating hepatitis C-infected inmates. As we show in Table 6, BOP's hepatitis C medication expenditures increased by almost 132 percent from fiscal year 2011 to 2012. FDA approved additional new medications at the end of 2013 and in 2014 that essentially cure hepatitis C, but that also drove up BOP's treatment costs. As these latest medications became the standard of care for treating hepatitis C, BOP was therefore required to use them. Table 6 also shows that BOP experienced an increase in hepatitis C medication expenditures of about 136 percent from fiscal year 2014 to 2015. Overall, BOP experienced an increase of about 427 percent for hepatitis C medication during the 8-year time period.[41] According to BOP officials, the average cost to treat one inmate

---

[39] Before adjusting for inflation, per capita pharmaceutical obligations increased from $357 per inmate in fiscal year 2009 to $715 per inmate in fiscal year 2016, or an increase of just over 100 percent.

[40] Biological products include a wide range of products such as vaccines, blood and blood components, allergenics, somatic cells, gene therapy, tissues, and recombinant therapeutic proteins. In contrast to most drugs that are chemically synthesized and their structure is known, most biologics are complex mixtures that are not easily identified or characterized.

[41] The Department of Veterans Affairs (VA) has also experienced these types of increases to treat hepatitis C, as our prior work has shown. See for example: GAO, *VA's Health Care Budget: In Response to a Projected Funding Gap in Fiscal Year 2015, VA Has Made Efforts to Better Manage Future Budgets*, GAO-16-584 (Washington, D.C.: June 3, 2016), and *VA's*

with the new medication ranges from $30,000 to $60,000. BOP treated 240 inmates in fiscal year 2015 and 327 inmates in fiscal year 2016 with the new medications. Additionally, according to BOP's 2018 Congressional Budget Justification, BOP estimated that there were approximately 20,000 inmates infected with hepatitis C, most of whom had not been treated. Table 6 also shows increases in expenditures for medication to treat cancer and HIV/AIDS. Overall, expenditures for cancer medication increased by about 315 percent during the 8 year time period, and by about 87 percent for HIV/AIDS medication.

Table 6. Bureau of Prisons' (BOP) pharmaceutical expenditures for hepatitis C, cancer, HIV/AIDS, and psychotropic drugs and percentage change from fiscal years 2009 through 2016

(Expenditures in millions of dollars, and percentage change in percentage)								
	Fiscal year							
	2009	2010	2011	2012	2013	2014	2015	2016
Hepatitis C medication expenditures	$2.6	$2.0	$1.9	$4.5	$4.2	$5.3	$12.6	$13.6
Hepatitis C medication percentage change from previous year	-	-24.6	-1.2	131.9	-6.4	27.1	136.3	8.7
Cancer medication expenditures	$1.9	$1.6	$2.1	$4.1	$3.7	$5.9	$6.4	$7.9
Cancer medication percentage change from previous year	-	-15.1	32.0	92.6	-10.4	60.3	7.8	24.3
HIV/AIDS medication expenditures	$14.6	$14.5	$16.1	$19.0	$20.1	$23.2	$25.1	$27.4
HIV/AIDS medication percentage change from previous year	-	-0.9	11.0	17.7	6.0	15.4	8.1	9.3
Psychotropic medication expenditures	$10.6	$10.2	$8.0	$7.0	$6.3	$4.2	$3.8	$2.7
Psychotropic medication percentage change from previous year	-	-2.9	-21.8	-12.2	-9.8	-33.1	-9.5	-29.1

Source: GAO analysis of BOP data. | GAO-17-379.

Note: These expenditures are based on BOP's annual list of top 50 medication expenditures and do not encompass the totality of expenditures on medications. On average, the top 50 medications make up about 67 percent of total pharmaceutical expenditures.

Health Care Budget: Preliminary Observations on Efforts to Improve Tracking of Obligations and Projected Utilization, GAO-16-374T (Washington, D.C.: Feb. 10, 2016).

To ensure appropriate management of the hepatitis C infected inmate population, BOP developed treatment criteria, consistent with the American Association for the Study of Liver Diseases guidelines, to expediently identify and treat inmates with the highest medical need.[42] In addition, the BOP Chief Pharmacist and other officials told us that they seek opportunities to acquire voluntary price reductions below the statutory Federal Supply Schedule pricing for hepatitis C medication from drug manufacturers.[43]

BOP data show that while pharmaceutical expenditures have increased overall, pharmaceutical expenditures for certain categories have varied, as can be seen in Table 6 and Figure 4. Expenditures have increased for hepatitis C, cancer, and HIV/AIDS medication, but decreased for psychotropic medications, which are generally used to treat mental health conditions. According to BOP officials, the availability of generic equivalents has helped decrease costs of psychotropic medication. Our prior work has also shown that generic drug prices have fallen overall since 2010, despite some extraordinary price increases in some generic medications.[44]

---

[42] The American Association for the Study of Liver Diseases (AASLD) is the leading organization of scientists and health care professionals committed to preventing and curing liver disease. AASLD develops evidence-based guidelines, which include recommendations of preferred approaches to the diagnostic, therapeutic, and preventative aspects of care related to liver disease.

[43] The Federal Supply Schedules (FSS) program, managed by the General Services Administration, provides federal agencies a simplified method of purchasing commercial products and services at prices associated with volume buying. A schedule is a set of contracts awarded to multiple vendors that provide similar products and services. BOP seeks price reductions to obtain a price lower than the FSS price, in accordance with Federal Acquisition Regulation 8.405-4, 48 C.F.R. § 8.405-4.

[44] See for example, GAO, *Generic Drugs Under Medicare: Part D Generic Drug Prices Declined Overall, but Some Had Extraordinary Price Increases*, GAO-16-706 (Washington, D.C.: Aug. 12, 2016), and *Prescription Drugs: Trends in Usual and Customary Prices for Commonly Used Drugs*, GAO-11-306R (Washington, D.C.: Feb. 10, 2011). Department of Health and Human Services, Office of the Assistant Secretary for Planning and Evaluation, *Understanding Recent Trends in Generic Drug Prices* (Washington, D.C.: Jan. 27, 2016).

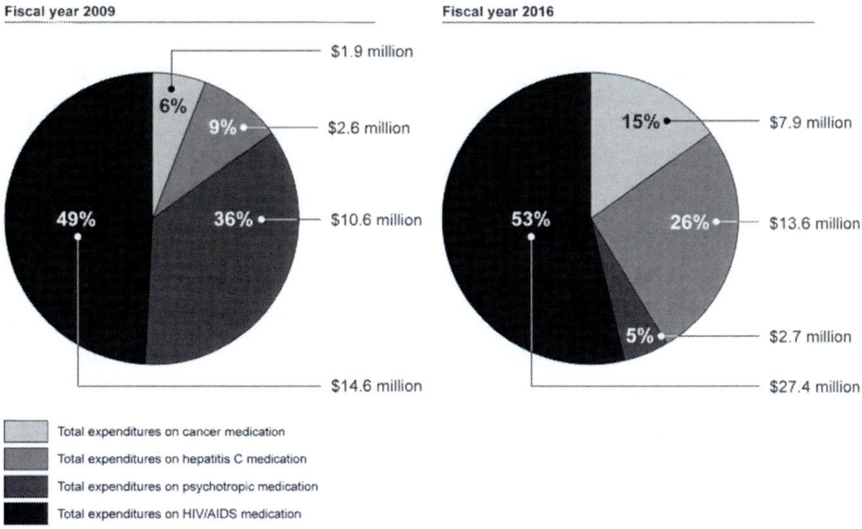

Source: GAO analysis of BOP data. | GAO-17-379.

Notes: Numbers may not total because of rounding.

These expenditures are based on BOP's annual list of top 50 medication expenditures and do not encompass the totality of expenditures on medications. On average, the top 50 medications make up about 67 percent of total pharmaceutical expenditures.

Figure 4. Change in Composition of Bureau of Prisons' (BOP) Expenditures for Hepatitis C, Cancer, HIV/AIDS, and Psychotropic Medication from Fiscal Years 2009 to 2016.

Outside Medical Services

BOP officials told us that costs for outside medical services have risen, which is another factor that is likely affecting their total obligations. According to BOP data, the total amount obligated increased from $322.6 million in fiscal year 2009 to $456.7 million in fiscal year 2016 (see Table 7), which is an increase of about 45 percent over this period.

As previously discussed, BOP incurs costs for outside care when BOP staff take inmates outside for specialty care that cannot be provided inside the institution, or for acute or emergency care, which could potentially become a catastrophic case.[45] We asked BOP for the catastrophic care cost

[45] BOP defines a catastrophic case as an event where an inmate in a medical care level 1, 2, or 3 institution incurs outside care costs of $35,000 or more, in conjunction with one of these

data for the 6 regions, for fiscal years 2014 and 2015. BOP was able to provide us the data for five of six regions for fiscal year 2015, and provided incomplete data for 2014 for most regions. When we asked one region why the data were incomplete, we were told that there was no requirement to collect such data. Although these data are incomplete, they show that BOP estimated costs of at least $100 million in fiscal year 2015 for catastrophic care in 5 of its 6 regions, which represents about 22 percent of outside medical services obligations for 2015. In its Congressional Budget Justifications from fiscal years 2009 through 2016, BOP reported that it had developed a process for monitoring and tracking catastrophic care costs; however, BOP officials acknowledged that their efforts to date have not been successful. During the course of our review, BOP designed a data collection instrument, which BOP officials stated they distributed to the regional offices, in order to more uniformly collect catastrophic care data moving forward.

Table 7. Bureau of Prisons' (BOP) outside medical services obligations from fiscal years 2009 through 2016 (in millions of dollars)

	Fiscal year							
	2009	2010	2011	2012	2013	2014	2015	2016
Outside medical services[a]	$322.6	$355.2	$366.1	$382.7	$419.9	$433.9	$453.2	$467.7
Percentage change from previous year	-	10.1	3.1	4.5	9.7	3.3	4.4	3.2

Source: GAO analysis of BOP data. | GAO-17-379.

[a]Outside medical services include obligations for contractual services related to the provision of health care.

Outside medical services made up about 40 percent of medical services obligations annually from fiscal years 2009 through 2016. According to BOP officials, BOP has difficulties attracting sufficient medical staff to

three events: requires a hospital stay of 7 days or more; has a hospital readmission within 30 days of discharge for the same diagnosis; or has a recurring medical need such as dialysis for kidney failure.

care for inmates in-house for institutions in remote locations, and therefore relies on outside care to a greater extent in these locations. We have also reported that BOP finds it particularly challenging to hire medical staff for institutions in rural locations because of the institutions' location and low pay in these areas.[46] In addition to the challenges posed by rural locations, some BOP institutions also have fewer community health care resources in proximity. As shown in Figure 5, we found that of the 98 BOP institutions, 64 of them have five or fewer hospitals within a 20 mile radius, and 9 had no hospitals within a 20 mile radius.[47] BOP officials also noted that the existence of a hospital in proximity to a BOP institution does not guarantee the hospital is willing to contract with BOP to serve an inmate population.[48] A DOJ OIG report found that in one BOP complex, a decline in staffing from fiscal year 2010 to fiscal year 2014 corresponded with an increase in outside medical services costs of 47 percent during the same period.[49] According to BOP officials, this is the primary reason BOP instituted its medical care level classification system, so the level of inmate health needs are matched to locations where community health care resources are sufficient.

---

[46] See GAO, *Bureau of Prisons: Management of New Prison Activations Can Be Improved*, GAO-14-709 (Washington, D.C.: Aug. 22, 2014). In this report, we found that BOP was encountering obstacles with hiring sufficient staff during the process of activating institutions, the process by which it prepares them for inmates, and therefore recommended that BOP analyze staffing data at individual institutions in the activation process to assess their progress toward reaching authorized staffing levels. BOP implemented this recommendation by September 2016.

[47] BOP has 122 BOP-operated institutions, 39 of which are located in one of 15 FCCs. FCCs are a cluster of institutions with different missions (for example, medical/mental health, pretrial, and holdover), which are located together. Because they are located together, for the purposes of this analysis we counted an FCC as one institution. When counting an FCC as one institution, there are 98 BOP institutions. We used 98 BOP institutions as the total number of institutions for our analysis.

[48] BOP officials stated that hospitals are not obligated to enter into contractual arrangements with BOP and some refuse due to concerns, such as not wanting inmates in their waiting rooms or entering through their front doors.

[49] DOJ OIG, *Review of the Federal Bureau of Prisons' Medical Staffing Challenges*, Evaluations and Inspections Division 16-02 (Washington, D.C.: March 2016).

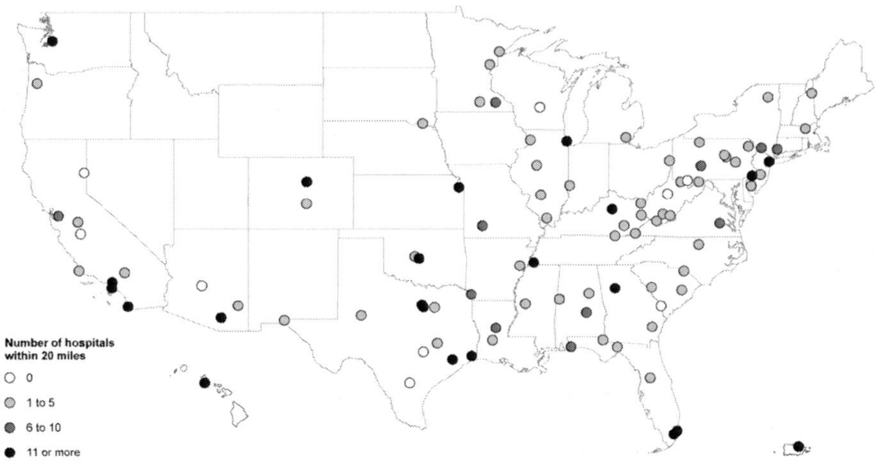

Source: GAO analysis of BOP data; MapInfo (map). | GAO-17-379.

Figure 5. Bureau of Prisons' (BOP) Institutions and Number of Hospitals within 20 Miles.

BOP Lacks or Does Not Analyze Certain Health Care Data Necessary to Understand and Control its Costs

BOP Lacks Health Care Utilization Data

BOP lacks data on the health care services it provides to inmates, which is otherwise known as health care utilization data.[50] BOP officials explained that existing data systems, such as the Financial Management Information System (FMIS), the accounting system of record, and BEMR, are not capable of collecting health care utilization data. Specifically, BOP cannot collect any health care utilization data from FMIS, because it is a DOJ-wide system and was not designed to allow DOJ components, such as BOP, to customize it. For example, while FMIS tracks expenditures on

[50] Utilization can be measured as the number of services provided to a patient, such as the number of X-rays. More often, however, a variety of procedures and services are of interest, and some measure of "cost" is assigned to each service so that resource intensity can be summed over all provided services.

categories such as salaries and supplies, it cannot be customized to analyze health care data. BOP officials also said they cannot collect financial data from BEMR because BEMR was not designed to collect such data.

BOP officials acknowledged that health care utilization data is important to understand and control health care costs, but recognized that BOP does not have data on its own use of resources. Officials also told us that BOP's lack of health care utilization data has stalled its implementation of one health care cost control opportunity identified in 2012 that would leverage its volume purchasing power while contracting for medical services. Specifically, BOP is planning to pilot a regional comprehensive medical services contract. However, according to BOP officials, they need to provide information to the potential contractors such as how utilization rates compare across institutions within the region, and across the different regions, in order for potential contractors to build proposals.[51] Because BOP is not positioned to provide utilization data, it cannot move forward with its plans. BOP officials also stated that a lack of data on its utilization of services stifles their ability to evaluate various health care cost control efforts.

Given these limitations, BOP has explored and identified some solutions since 2009 to collect data on its utilization of health care services but has not yet determined how to obtain health care utilization data.[52] Examples include the following:

- In fiscal year 2009, BOP began utilizing a medical claims adjudication services contract through which BOP sought, in part, to gather data on the utilization of health services outside its institutions.[53] While BOP officials stated they intended to

---

[51] Generally, each BOP institution has its own contract for outside medical services. Under the proposed regional pilot, BOP would award a single regional comprehensive medical services contract to cover health care for all BOP institutions in one region. This could save the agency $30 million per year, according to internal BOP documents. However, BOP did not have any documentation of the analysis underlying this estimate.

[52] GAO did not evaluate the solutions BOP described to determine whether they would achieve BOP's objectives.

[53] The primary objective of medical claims adjudication was to ensure compliance with the applicable negotiated fee schedule for medical services. BOP requires that its medical

eventually cover all BOP institutions under this contract, as of February 2017, only 23 BOP institutions have used the service. BOP officials explained that BOP did not add more institutions to the initial medical claims adjudication contract because the contract ended before it could do so. BOP officials could not explain why more institutions had not utilized the services in the five years preceding the end of the contract, but some regional officials we spoke with, and officials at some of the institutions we visited, said the medical claims adjudication services provided were not cost effective. Senior BOP officials disagreed with the regional officials' statement and said that the services were necessary to verify that medical services invoices were correct. BOP created a solicitation for a new contract in February 2016, and, as of February 2017, BOP was evaluating offers. According to officials, BOP is reviewing several proposals to contract for medical claims adjudication services for all BOP-managed institutions and expects to award the contract in early spring 2017.

- In fiscal year 2016, BOP contracted for a study to consider various options to enhance its ability to collect and analyze data through BEMR, including data on utilization of health care services inside and outside BOP's institutions. The study considered three options— keeping the existing system as is, enhancing the existing system, or replacing the system entirely. The study included costs and recommendations for BOP to consider. As of February 2017, BOP officials indicated that they are still exploring these options.
- In fiscal year 2016, to provide potential vendors with utilization data to pilot the regional comprehensive health care contract, as described earlier, BOP began searching for computer software to convert its paper claims for outside medical services into electronic format files. Such files would include the inmate's description, the condition for treatment, the service provided, and the cost of treatment. As of February 2017, BOP officials had not yet

claims adjudication services provider also make data available on a periodic and as needed basis.

identified any cost-effective solutions through which to convert paper claims but said they continue to pursue this option.

In fiscal year 2016, BOP officials also attempted to devise a method to collect health care utilization data from each of its institutions; however, they did not implement this approach after receiving feedback from institution-based personnel that it would be too burdensome on them to implement. As of February 2017, according to officials, BOP continues to explore options to collect and analyze utilization data based on the experiences of other health care systems. For example, BOP convened a federal interagency group to discuss how other federal agencies study utilization rates and discussed with officials from the California Department of Corrections the approach those officials have taken.

BOP officials recognize the importance of finding a solution to collect utilization data and has identified, and in some cases attempted then abandoned, various possible solutions. However, BOP officials told us that they were not aware of OMB guidance on how to conduct a cost-effectiveness analysis, which describes how to systematically evaluate options, and would review it as they continue to pursue a solution to BOP's lack of utilization data.[54] OMB Circular A-94 calls for conducting a cost-effectiveness analysis when the benefits from competing alternatives are the same or where a policy decision has been made that the benefits must be provided.[55] By conducting a cost-effectiveness analysis of the potential ways to obtain health care utilization data, BOP will be better positioned to determine the most cost-effective way to collect such data and to start doing so in a timely manner.

---

[54] OMB defines cost-effectiveness as a systematic quantitative method for comparing the costs of alternative means of achieving the same stream of benefits or a given objective. OMB, *Guidelines and Discount Rates for Benefit-Cost Analysis of Federal Programs*, Circular No. A-94 (Washington, D.C.: Oct. 29, 1992).

[55] OMB, Circular A-94, *Guidelines and Discount Rates for Benefit-Cost Analysis of Federal Programs*. OMB Circular A-94 provides guidance for cost-effectiveness analyses. Cost-Effectiveness analysis is a less comprehensive technique than a benefit-cost analysis but can be appropriate when considering competing alternatives with the same benefit.

BOP Does Not Analyze Available Health Care Spending Data

BOP has not consistently collected and analyzed its institutions' health care spending data to identify additional cost control opportunities, such as through strategic sourcing. Strategic sourcing is a process that moves an organization away from numerous individual procurements toward a broader, aggregate procurement approach. This broader approach generally begins with an analysis of spending (spend analysis) and the identification of products and services for which a more effective sourcing strategy could be implemented.[56] We have emphasized the importance of conducting a comprehensive spend analysis for strategic sourcing purposes since 2002. The approach provides knowledge about how much is being spent for goods and services, who the buyers are, who the suppliers are, and where the opportunities are to save money and improve performance.[57]

BOP officials told us that they do not routinely analyze or review BOP's spending data to identify new opportunities for cost savings through strategic sourcing. BOP procurement officials told us they search for strategic sources for a health care good or service once their colleagues in HSD notify them that BOP needs to obtain the good or service. BOP officials told us it is time intensive to collect and analyze spending data. Nevertheless, they acknowledged the benefits of strategic sourcing and stated they need to seek additional strategic sourcing opportunities. In fiscal year 2013, BOP identified health care supplies/services as a target area for identifying cost savings opportunities that are likely to produce significant savings through strategic sourcing. Further, according to BOP's April 2016 Strategic Sourcing Program guidance, the key to the strategic sourcing program is a thorough analysis of spending patterns— or a spend

---

[56] OMB defines strategic sourcing as the collaborative and structured process of critically analyzing an organization's spending and using this information to make business decisions about acquiring commodities and services more effectively and efficiently. OMB, *Memorandum for Chief Acquisition Officers, Chief Financial Officers, and Chief Information Officers on Implementing Strategic Sourcing* (Washington, D.C.: 2005).

[57] GAO, *Strategic Sourcing: Leading Commercial Practices Can Help Federal Agencies Increase Savings When Acquiring Services*, GAO-13-417 (Washington, D.C.: Apr. 15, 2013). See also, *Best Practices: Using Spend Analysis to Help Agencies Take a More Strategic Approach to Procurement*, GAO-04-870 (Washington, D.C.: Sept. 16, 2004).

analysis—to determine what is being purchased, how it is being purchased, the dollar value of those purchases, and which vendors are involved. This guidance is consistent with GAO's prior work on leading commercial practices in strategic sourcing.[58] However, despite this guidance, BOP officials told us that they had not yet reviewed health care spending data and could not identify any BOP official who would have the time to complete the task.

Although BOP has not conducted a spend analysis, it has identified and implemented some strategic sourcing opportunities, such as pursuing national contracts so that all institutions can pay for the same goods or services at the same negotiated rates. When national contracts are not in place, each BOP institution generally procures health care goods and services on an individual basis and some institutions have individually procured the same medical care equipment or services at varied costs. For example, several institutions have either purchased or leased one particular brand of robotic equipment to dispense medication as part of their pharmaceutical operations, but costs for the equipment varied across the institutions—one had an initial purchase cost of about $122,000, while another had an initial annual lease cost that was about $43,000. BOP officials also told us that they identify strategic sourcing opportunities through discussions with other agencies and have participated in interagency collaboration on strategic sourcing.

According to BOP documentation, BOP does not have a single data system that can provide health care spending data for a spend analysis; however, existing sources, such as the Federal Procurement Data System-Next Generation (FPDS-NG), could assist BOP in its data collection effort. For example, BOP records all contracts with estimated values above a certain threshold (currently $3,500) in the FPDS-NG, a database used by agencies across the federal government to record procurement information.[59] Additionally, according to BOP officials, each institution's

---

[58] GAO-13-417.

[59] FPDS-NG can be accessed at https://www.fpds.gov. FPDS-NG data and reporting requirements for FPDS-NG are described in FAR subpart 4.6, 48 C.F.R. subpart 4.6. The micro-purchase threshold became $3,500 in July 2015. 80 Fed. Reg. 38, 293, 38, 294 (July 2, 2015) (codified at 48 C.F.R. § 2.101).

business administrators regularly audit spending data from purchase cards—cards used by government agencies to buy goods or services. One BOP region, for example, created a method to monitor its institutions' spending through its local accounting program that helped the region identify opportunities to control costs. Officials found, when they began tracking some aspects of institutional spending, that two institutions within that region were spending \$5,000-\$10,000 more per year on biohazardous waste disposal than other institutions. As a result, officials from the region contacted the institutions' management and asked them to identify lower cost vendors, which the institutions did. Conducting spend analyses using these existing and readily available data sources could provide BOP with several benefits, including knowledge about how much is being spent for given products and services, who the buyers and suppliers are, and where opportunities exist for BOP to use strategic sourcing to leverage buying and save money.

BOP Has Initiatives Aimed to Control Health Care Costs but Has Not Assessed Their Effectiveness, Applied a Sound Planning Approach, or Documented its Analyses of Federal Medical Centers' Missions

BOP Has Initiatives Intended to Control Health Care Costs but Has Not Evaluated Their Effectiveness

BOP-Wide Initiatives

BOP has taken bureau-wide actions to help control health care costs through several initiatives, but has generally not evaluated the effectiveness of these initiatives. We reviewed BOP documents to identify initiatives aimed at health care cost control for the period beginning with fiscal year 2009 through November 2016. Through our review and discussions with BOP officials, as of February 2017, we found that BOP had 10 initiatives aimed at controlling its health care costs (see Table 8).[60] The table provides a description of each initiative and status.

Table 8. Bureau of Prisons (BOP)-identified health care costs savings initiatives from fiscal years (FY) 2009 through February 2017

Initiative, with year implemented	BOP Description
Implemented	
1. Pharmaceutical Procurement [2008]	BOP participates in initiatives to leverage the combined purchase requirements with the Department of Veterans Affairs, Department of Defense and Indian Health Service. Additionally the BOP seeks opportunities to acquire voluntary price reductions from manufacturers below statutory Federal Supply Schedule pricing.[a]
2. Pharmaceuticals Prime Vendor Program [2000]	The Pharmaceuticals Prime Vendor Program enables BOP to leverage high volume purchasing to reduce the individual pricing of select medications.
3. Contract Dental Lab Operations [2009]	The BOP dental program provides prosthetics to inmate patients that are partially or completely toothless. Dental laboratory services are provided by the national contracted vendor when one is available.
Partially Implemented	
4. Bill Adjudication (Medical Claims Adjudication) [est. FY2009]	BOP contracts with a medical claims adjudication vendor to review claims for duplicate billing, claims for services not requested or not appropriate for the stated diagnoses, and local market rates for physician and facility charges in 23 BOP institutions (as of February 2017). Contracting for medical claims adjudication enables BOP to identify patterns of fraud, waste, and abuse. BOP plans to fully implement this initiative in its remaining institutions once a new contract is awarded.
5. National Contracts for Medical Resources [FY2017]	BOP signed an Interagency Agreement with the Department of Veteran Affairs to use its Medical/Surgical Prime Vendor Program, which allows BOP institutions to purchase medical and surgical supplies. According to BOP officials, this initiative is currently in the start-up phase.

[60] BOP initially provided several more health care cost control initiatives but BOP officials later determined that only 10 were health care cost control initiatives. BOP officials told us that during the course of this review, they determined that the other initiatives were aimed at clinical care or administrative reporting, rather than cost control.

Table 8. (Continued)

Initiative, with year implemented	BOP Description
6. Equipment Standardization [FY2017]	BOP's Health Services Division (HSD) is in the process of updating its enterprise Automated Inventory Management System to standardize major medical equipment.
Planned	
7. Regional Comprehensive Medical Services Contracts [est. implementation in FY2020]	BOP is exploring the feasibility of regional comprehensive medical services contracts that serve a multi-state area. Currently, BOP institutions use separate contracts.
8. Federal Ceiling Price (Big 4 Pricing) for Pharmaceuticals [est. implementation unknown][b]	BOP is currently not included in the federal law that establishes the Federal Ceiling Price (Big 4 Pricing) for pharmaceuticals. As a result, BOP often pays more for pharmaceuticals than other government agencies. According to BOP officials, BOP is exploring the feasibility of legislation being passed to make Big 4 pricing available to BOP.
9. BOP Mail Order Pharmacy (BOPMOP) [est. implementation within 5 years]	BOPMOP is an initiative that is to enable remotely located pharmacists to receive automated orders from BOP institutions for dispensing prescribed medications and mailing the packaged medications to the inmate needing pharmaceutical therapy. The remote fill operation will replace the need for hiring/retaining an on-site pharmacist in institutions that house mostly healthy inmates, and provides temporary back-up for institutions experiencing a prolonged absence of an institution pharmacist (e.g., due to an extended illness). BOP officials believe that BOPMOP will maximize pharmacy resources by consolidating storage of prescription drugs into one central inventory and through buying the least expensive brand of generic medications.
Planned	
10. Unit Dose Repackaging [unknown]	BOP plans to purchase bulk medication, which is generally less expensive than purchasing unit dose packaged items, and repackage them locally or at a central location.

Source: GAO analysis of BOP data. | GAO-17-379.

Note: For the purpose of this report, we included initiatives that began prior to fiscal year 2009 if they continued to be implemented during the period of fiscal year 2009 to November 2016.

[a]The Federal Supply Schedules (FSS) program, managed by the General Services Administration, provides federal agencies a simplified method of purchasing commercial products and services at prices associated with volume buying. A schedule is a set of contracts awarded to multiple vendors that provide similar products and services. According to officials, BOP seeks price reductions to obtain a price lower than the FSS price, in accordance with Federal Acquisition Regulation 8.405-4, 48 C.F.R. § 8.405-4.

[b]Federal ceiling prices, also called Big Four prices, are available to the Departments of Veterans Affairs and Defense, the Public Health Service, and the U.S. Coast Guard. These prices are mandated by law to be lower than nonfederal average manufacturer prices.

BOP had also reported six other cost containment initiatives or systems in its fiscal year 2017 Congressional Budget Justification. BOP officials explained that although they had previously publicly reported that these initiatives were designed to contain health care costs, during the course of our review they realized that their primary purpose was instead for clinical or administrative purposes. BOP officials stated that there may be a secondary gain of cost avoidance, but regardless of cost avoidance, they would have carried out the initiatives. BOP reported these cost containment initiatives or systems again in its fiscal year 2018 Congressional Budget Justification (see Table 9).

Table 9. Bureau of Prisons (BOP) health care costs savings initiatives as reported in fiscal year 2018 congressional budget justification

Initiative, with year implemented	BOP Description
Implemented	
1. Telehealth [2004][a]	BOP uses telehealth for the following: to conduct specialty medicine clinics in some federal medical centers; to deliver specialty medical services to remote locations; to provide psychiatric services and manage psychotropic medications; to consult with institutions on dermatological cases to assess need for community services versus onsite care; to consult with institutions on dietetics and diabetes; to allow regional staff to conduct chronic care visits in their regional institutions; and to facilitate chronic care and follow-up visits across facilities in BOP complexes.
2. Levels of Care [2004]	BOP assigns each inmate and each BOP facility a care level (i.e., care level 1 = essentially healthy; care level 2 = stable chronic conditions; care level 3 = chronic conditions with manageable complications; care level 4 = need for continuous nursing care). BOP reported that this medical classification system enables it to allot its resources to better manage inmates' medical and mental health needs.
3. Utilization Review [2009]	BOP requires every institution to implement a utilization review process to assure that only medically necessary care is provided. Health care staff use an automated utilization review program for clinical decision-making criteria that aims to differentiate between what is medically necessary from what is potentially elective care.

Table 9. (Continued)

Initiative, with year implemented	BOP Description
4. Catastrophic Case Management [2012][b]	BOP institutions and regional offices monitor cases of hospitalized inmates and track catastrophic costs to closely manage care and expedite inmate transfers to BOP medical centers when feasible.
5. National Pharmacy & Therapeutics Committee [1996]	BOP's National Pharmacy & Therapeutics Committee researches drug efficacy and safety, and manages a tightly controlled National Drug Formulary that favors generic drugs.[c]
Partially Implemented	
6. Electronic Medical Records System (Health Information Technologies) [FY2008]	BOP-wide deployment of a base electronic medical record was completed in fiscal year 2008. The Bureau Electronic Medical Record system (BEMR) includes the components of the traditional health record, with a prescription component. It utilizes secure wireless technology to bring health care documentation to the patient's bedside on nursing care units and any other area in BOP facilities where care is provided (i.e., special housing units). BOP noted that it planned to integrate a Laboratory Information System that collects information from BOP's medical laboratories with BEMR, continue to refine processes, and add ancillary documentation components in compliance with the Office of the National Coordinator for Health Information Technology's standards.[d]

Source: GAO analysis of BOP data. | GAO-17-379.

[a]Telehealth is the use of electronic information and telecommunications technologies to support long distance clinical health care, patient and professional health related education, public health and health administration. See Health Resources and Services Administration "Telehealth."

[b]While BOP institutions and regional offices monitor cases of hospitalized inmates as they occur, BOP Central Office does not systematically track catastrophic care costs over time, and did not require the regions to collect this information. GAO requested BOP's catastrophic data for fiscal years 2014-2015 but the data were incomplete. In 2016, BOP created a template for its regions to collect catastrophic care costs in a more systematic way. This effort remains in progress.

[c]The national formulary is a list of medications that can be prescribed and dispensed by BOP clinicians without additional authorization from higher-level officials. The National Pharmacy & Therapeutics Committee meets regularly to review the national formulary.

[d]The Department of Health and Human Services' Office of the National Coordinator for Health Information Technology is responsible for overseeing the certification of electronic health record (EHR) technology, including establishing EHR technical standards and certification criteria.

Of the 16 initiatives BOP either identified for us (Table 8), or reported in its fiscal year 2018 Congressional Budget Justification (Table 9), BOP could only provide documentation for 1 cost savings estimate, as we show in Table 10. BOP provided documentation demonstrating the analysis for its estimated cost savings for the initiative to contract for its dental lab operations.[61] BOP officials stated that BOP does not have a process to evaluate cost savings and that evaluating all of its initiatives would be very labor intensive. BOP officials also told us that they can sometimes assume cost savings. For example, BOP implemented a system of medical and mental health care levels for its institutions and inmates to match health care needs to health care resources. According to BOP officials, the cost control results of this initiative can be assumed; however, in internal BOP documentation, officials acknowledge that although the system was designed to reduce cost, its results are undetermined. BOP officials stated that BOP does not have an automated data system to collect and analyze cost savings data in this manner.

Table 10. Bureau of Prisons (BOP) health care cost savings initiatives with cost savings estimates (fiscal year 2009 through November 2016)

Number of Initiatives		Number of Initiatives with Documented Cost Savings Estimates
Implemented	8	1[a]
Partially Implemented	4	0
Planned	4	0
Total	16	1

Source: GAO analysis of BOP data. GAO-17-379.

[a]BOP provided documentation for its estimated cost savings for the initiative to transition dental lab operations to an outside vendor.

BOP had previously developed a process for collecting and analyzing cost data without automated data systems. Specifically, In 2011, in response to a DOJ OIG recommendation, BOP reported to the OIG that it had established a four-step process to collect and analyze data to determine the cost-effectiveness of current and future health care cost control

[61] BOP provided its methodology for estimating cost savings for three planned cost savings initiatives—Federal Ceiling (Big 4) Price, BOPMOP, and Unit Dose Repackaging—but did not provide documentation of analysis to support its cost savings estimate.

initiatives for which BOP has or can collect data.[62] As part of the process, BOP reported that it would implement the following four steps: (1) generate an initiative for HSD and/or BOP executive staff approval; (2) identify factors to measure an approved initiative's outcomes and establish benchmarks; (3) capture relevant and available program and cost data (to the extent possible using existing data systems) on at least an annual basis; and (4) analyze the data and produce cost-benefit reports for HSD leadership. At that time, BOP listed seven initiatives it could evaluate using this process, and it provided evidence to the OIG that it had used this process to evaluate one of those seven initiatives. As a result, an OIG official told us the OIG closed the recommendation. However, BOP officials told us they have not continued to use this process to determine the cost-effectiveness of its initiatives, and do not have a process in place to determine the cost-effectiveness of its initiatives. When we asked BOP officials about the process, as described to the OIG, they told us that they were unaware of its existence until we inquired about its use. *Standards for Internal Control in the Federal Government* calls for management to design control activities to achieve its objectives, including evaluations to compare actual performance to planned or expected results.[63] By regularly evaluating health care cost control initiatives for which it has or can collect data, BOP would be better positioned to determine if the time and resources it is investing to control costs has been effective, or whether it should alter its path to achieve better outcomes.

Regional and Institutional Initiatives

Some of BOP's regions and institutions have also undertaken various initiatives that officials described as having a cost control impact. BOP officials told us that regions and institutions make decisions about whether and which initiatives to implement based on institutions' varied needs and circumstances. For example, BOP encourages institutions to use contract

---

[62] U.S. Department of Justice Office of Inspector General, *The Federal Bureau Of Prisons' Efforts To Manage Inmate Health Care*, Audit Division 08-08 (Washington, D.C.: February 2008).

[63] GAO, *Standards for Internal Control in the Federal Government*, GAO-14-704G (Washington, D.C.: Sep. 10, 2014).

guards, rather than BOP correctional officers, to supervise inmates during treatment in community medical facilities. According to BOP officials from some institutions we visited, the use of contract guards can result in cost savings when compared to overtime costs paid to salaried correctional officers.[64] However, some institution officials told us that security concerns and emergent medical conditions affect their ability to use contract guards. In addition, officials from several of the institutions we visited said they reduce inmate custody and transportation costs by transporting inmates in groups by bus when they require outside health care. An institution's ability to use busing may depend on inmates' medical needs or the willingness of community providers to accommodate several inmates, according to officials.

Additionally, within individual institutions, some BOP officials have developed innovative cost control initiatives. For example, one official in an institution we visited said he had created metrics to measure and manage health care costs, including pharmaceutical costs, as well as the number of outside medical trips, and outside medical service costs, and then successfully took action to quantify reductions across all three. Also, one regional official said he created a mobile ophthalmology clinic to provide specialty eye services to institutions throughout the region and estimated costs savings in service charges and custody costs for each visit. In another example, officials at one FMC we visited told us they expanded the physical therapy program in various ways to control costs. For example, the program offers its specialized staff to consult on cases in other institutions, utilizes unpaid physical therapy interns, and encourages its staff to specialize to perform procedures that would otherwise take place outside the institution, such as electromyography,[65] according to officials.[66]

---

[64] BOP did not have a cost savings estimate but institution officials noted lower overtime costs due to this practice.

[65] Electromyography is a diagnostic test to assess the health of muscles and the nerve cells that control them.

[66] BOP did not have documentation to demonstrate this cost savings but institution officials explained that these initiatives controlled the institution's health care costs.

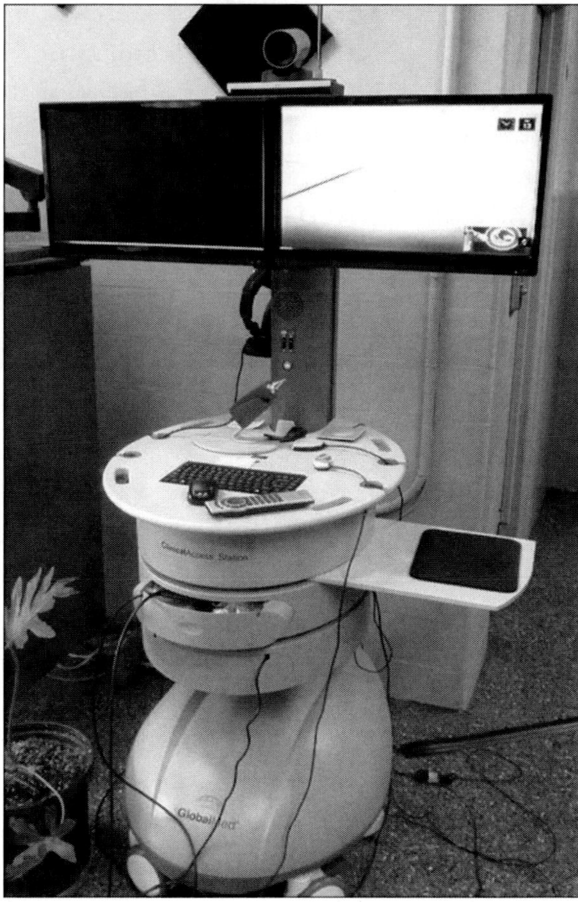

Source: BOP. | GAO-17-379.

Figure 6. Federal Medical Center Lexington Utilizes Specialized Telehealth Equipment to Conduct Specialty Clinics.

BOP institutions have also sought to use technology to control health care costs. Notably, officials at FMC Lexington said that they have a partnership with an outside medical services provider, which provides the institution with some advanced telehealth equipment (see Figure 6). This has allowed it to expand its use of telehealth to more than twenty medical specialties. For fiscal year 2015, FMC Lexington officials estimated a cost savings of over $1.5 million due to their use of telehealth. Many institutions have also sought to acquire other kinds of equipment to control health care costs. For example, some institutions have purchased or leased robotics to support their pharmaceutical operations (see Figure 7), which has reduced the burden on staff to manually fill prescriptions and improve operational efficiency. According to BOP officials, the use of robotics equipment in its institutions' pharmacies allows BOP pharmacists to devote more time to improving patient outcomes by providing clinical pharmacist services. Officials in another FMC we visited told us they purchased a pressure mapping system for the institution's wound program to identify and prevent ulcers, which institution officials estimate has saved nearly $2.8 million for the period covering fiscal year 2009 through 2015.

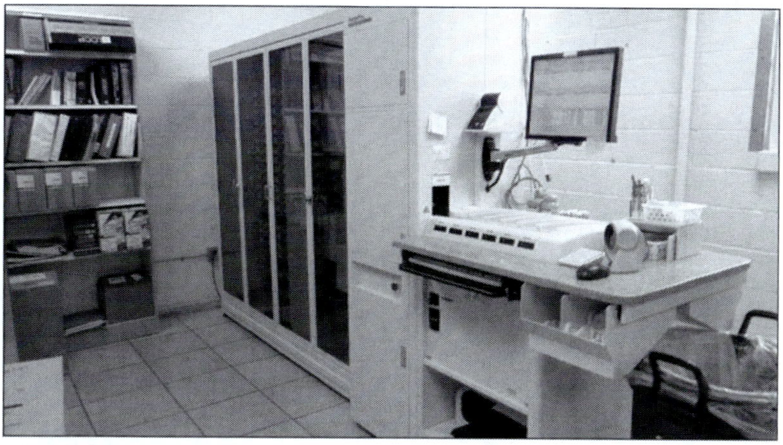

Source: BOP. | GAO-17-379.

Figure 7. Some Bureau of Prisons (BOP) Institutions Utilize Pharmacy Robotics to Reduce the Use of Manual Labor to Dispense Medication.

According to officials, institutions share and learn about one another's approaches to health care cost control through various platforms. For example, BOP compiles its institutions' reported cost efficiencies and innovations, including those related to health care, in a catalogue that is designed to be a reference to all institution managers regarding the activities of their peers. Institution officials also share information on health care cost control through regular conferences and meetings. For example, officials at one institution we visited stated that they employ the practice of having an institution nurse check on hospitalized inmates on a weekly basis to determine if they can return to the institution to complete their care in order to avoid custody and hospitalization costs. The officials using this practice said they presented it at a BOP symposium where officials from other institutions also presented their best health care practices. Officials also told us that as BOP officials transfer from one institution to another, they can also transfer information about health care cost control.

BOP Has Planned and Implemented Initiatives without Considering Certain Elements of Sound Planning

Table 11. Elements of sound planning applicable to GAO's assessment of the bureau of prisons' planning process

Elements	Description
Goals and objectives, activities, milestones, and performance measures	The identification of goals and objectives to be achieved by the plan, activities, or actions to achieve those results, as well as milestones to measure progress and performance measures to assess the effectiveness of activities.
Resources and investments	The identification of costs to execute the plan and the sources and types of resources and investments, including skills and technology and the human, capital, information, and other resources required to meet the goals and objectives.

Source: GAO. | GAO-17-379.

BOP's long-standing strategic planning process has focused in some part on health care cost control, but BOP's overall planning practices have not incorporated certain elements of sound planning that we have previously identified. These elements generally call for the identification of objectives with a means to measure (1) progress toward objectives and (2) the effectiveness of activities to achieve objectives. They also call for the identification of resources and investments (as shown in Table 11).[67]

[67] We selected these elements from GAO's body of work on sound planning based on their applicability to BOP documents and officials' statements on sound planning. GAO has also reported on other elements in sound planning, including the identification of a mission statement; problem, scope and methodology; integration among and with other entities;

As part of its annual BOP-wide strategic plans, BOP developed the HSD Cost Efficiency and Innovation strategic objective to "maximize health care resources as a cost-containment strategy by applying evidence-based business practices and measuring performance through the use of appropriate industry-wide metrics."[68] However, this objective does not include measures of effectiveness or progress, such as milestones or performance measures, which, when properly supported by reliable data, are critical to effectively measuring improvement. BOP established this objective in 2011 with six underlying activities it refers to as action plans. BOP officials told us that a strategic objective is considered achieved when the action plans are completed. However, simply completing an action plan does not ensure progress toward the achievement of the objective. For example, one of BOP's action plans under its HSD Cost Efficiency and Innovation strategic objective was to develop a methodology for ensuring health care expenditures reflect actual costs. BOP established nine metrics to evaluate financial performance and marked this action plan as "complete" in 2013. However, as of August 2016, BOP officials told us that they have not been able to collect comprehensive data for six of the nine metrics because of limitations to BOP's existing data systems or incomplete reporting. Moreover, BOP officials recognized the issues with this action because they stated that they are reconsidering the metrics they initially established. Thus, while BOP determined it had completed this action plan, the action itself did not produce any meaningful results. Although it is important for BOP to plan the actions or activities that it will take to achieve its objectives, it cannot rely only on the completion of activities to determine that it is achieving them. Without a means to measure progress toward its objective or effectiveness of its activities,

roles, responsibilities and coordination; key external factors. See GAO, *Executive Guide: Effectively Implementing the Government Performance and Results Act*, GAO/GGD-96-118 (Washington, D.C.: June 1996); *Combating Terrorism: Evaluation of Selected Characteristics in National Strategies Related to Terrorism*, GAO-04-408T (Washington, D.C.: Feb. 3, 2004); and *Veterans' Health Care: Proper Plan Needed to Modernize System for Paying Community Providers*, GAO-16-353 (Washington, D.C.: May 11, 2016).

[68] BOP changed the name of this objective in its 2015 BOP-wide strategic plan. It had been previously named "Healthcare Efficiency." There are other strategic objectives that relate to health care cost control, including Care Levels, BEMR, and Telehealth.

BOP cannot reliably determine whether it is achieving its objective or that its efforts are effective. Determining whether or not BOP is making progress toward its HSD Cost Efficiency and Innovation strategic objective and whether its efforts are effective will also allow BOP management to determine what midcourse corrections may be needed in order to meet the objective.

In addition to the annual BOP-wide strategic plan, HSD established a five- year HSD Integrated Strategic Plan for the period of 2015 through 2019, which applies a financial management focus to every HSD branch and section. The financial management goal, which is the same for every HSD branch and section, is to "effectively manage the Health Services budget through an ongoing analysis of staffing, program efficiencies, and utilization of services to identify opportunities for current and future cost containment." Although HSD includes the financial management goal for each HSD branch or section, as well as the branch or section's implementation strategies and expected outcomes, the expected outcomes are generally not measurable. For example, the description of the financial management goal for HSD's Health Services Branch is to "employ new strategies to contain health care costs while maintaining quality of services" and the expected outcome is "BOP health care costs are strategically contained." HSD does not indicate how it will measure progress toward its larger goal, and its expected outcome provides no means of measuring progress. By stating that it aims to contain costs strategically, but not including performance measures to assess the effectiveness of activities—HSD's planning efforts do not incorporate the elements of sound planning we have noted. Out of the 17 HSD branches and sections included in the HSD integrated strategic plan, only one—Pharmacy—included target benchmarks for financial management.

BOP officials told us that because BOP's per capita inmate health care costs are lower than the national health expenditure average per capita costs, BOP believes its efforts have successfully achieved cost savings. However, BOP's health care obligations exceeded $1.3 billion in fiscal year 2016, which is a significant portion of its nearly $6.9 billion appropriation, and its per capita health care obligations have continued to rise, particularly since 2013, which highlight the importance of controlling health care costs regardless of societal trends in health care spending.[69] Developing goals and objectives that include a means to measure progress would better position BOP management to assess its efforts to control health care costs and ensure these efforts are effective in achieving desired results.

As described previously, sound planning also calls for the identification of necessary resources and investments. BOP officials acknowledged that they do not systematically plan health care cost savings initiatives. As a result, BOP has not consistently identified the necessary resources and investments needed to implement its cost savings initiatives, or the external factors that could affect the achievement of its goals prior to implementation. For example, since 2011, BOP has planned to establish a mail-order or central fill pharmacy. BOP asserted that establishing a mail-order or central fill pharmacy would help it maximize pharmacy resources by consolidating prescription drugs into one main inventory.

BOP reported in its Congressional Budget Justification for fiscal year 2017 that this effort could save BOP $10 million per year in inventory costs.[70] To implement this initiative, BOP began restructuring its pharmaceutical operations at its care level 1 institutions, with plans to continue doing so with care level 2 institutions. Two years later, in 2013, BOP noted that the costs of this initiative would exceed available agency funding and BOP would have to request additional funding from the Congress to support the initiative. When we asked BOP officials why the initiative had not yet been implemented, they told us that in any given year when BOP sought to implement this initiative, it had either the funding or the space, but not both at the same time. Because BOP did not consider necessary resources and investments when this initiative was planned this initiative was not implemented earlier. Without consistently identifying the investments and resources needed, BOP risks expending unnecessary time

---

[69] The nearly $6.9 billion appropriation is for the Salaries and Expenses portion of BOP's fiscal year 2016 annual appropriation and does not include the separate Buildings and Facilities appropriation for fiscal year 2016.

[70] BOP provided its methodology for estimating the cost savings but did not have documentation for the analysis of this estimate.

and limited resources pursuing cost control initiatives that eventually may fail to achieve their goal of cost control.

BOP Does Not Document Its Mission Analyses of Its Federal Medical Centers

BOP employs a process every 3 to 4 years that it calls its "mission analysis," to assess how effectively the care it provides meet the needs of inmates having complex medical and mental health disorders in its FMCs. BOP officials told us that they make decisions about how to allocate resources based on mission analyses; however, BOP does not document these analyses and therefore lacks a record to support decision-making for its resource allocations. During mission analysis, BOP seeks to determine how effectively its health care programs, resources, and community-based services meet the needs of inmates, determine priorities, assess potential efficiencies, and make recommendations for change. To conduct a mission analysis, BOP also conducts a cost assessment, which officials described as including a review of outside medical trips, contracted services, elective procedures, and overtime for escorted medical trips to community-based facilities and providers. BOP officials stated that the cost analysis team also reviews relevant documents with the local staff responsible for these activities, and gives an oral report once it concludes its work. As a result of these mission analyses, BOP institutions have adjusted or added new health care programs. For example, FMC Butner officials stated that after a mission analysis was completed there, BOP saw the need for, and subsequently established, hospice care services. Also, according to BOP, the mission analysis can provide officials with the information needed to consolidate or shift resources from one care level 4 institution to another. BOP recently made this kind of shift in resources in December 2016 when it converted Federal Correctional Institution Fort Worth to a Federal Medical Center and has already requested 36 full-time equivalents and over $4.7 million to expand and renovate the facility.

When we asked BOP for more information on how they conduct the mission analysis process or examples of written materials that guided their decision making, BOP officials told us they only document what participants consider the highlights in an executive summary. For example, the 2016 mission analysis for FMC Rochester that BOP provided to us was an overview of its health care services and staffing, and recommendations for consideration. While the summary included recommendations, it did not include the analysis and findings to support the recommendations. BOP officials stated that the mission analysis was an opportunity for Central Office, region and institution leadership to meet and verbally discuss the status of the institution's missions, challenges, resources and ongoing activities. Nevertheless, Standards for *Internal Control in the Federal Government* calls for documentation as a necessary part of an effective internal control system, which is required to demonstrate its design, implementation and operating effectiveness.[71] Documenting its analyses and findings could help provide reasonable assurance that recommendations to shift resources at its higher care level institutions are based on sound evidence. According to BOP data, those higher care level institutions account for a sizable portion of medical services costs. Specifically, BOP's six care level 4 institutions—prior to adding Fort Worth to this list—accounted for about $350 million (or about 30 percent) of BOP's medical services costs for fiscal year 2015 while housing about seven percent of the inmate population.

CONCLUSION

Providing health care, including medical, dental, and mental health care, to the federal inmate population is an important and required part of BOP's broader mission to safely, humanely, and securely confine offenders in prisons. While BOP's inmate population has fallen since fiscal year 2014, health care costs have continued to increase in total, and on an

[71] GAO-14-704G.

annual per capita basis, due in part to factors that BOP cannot control, such as the aging inmate population, increasing pharmaceutical costs, and increasing costs of medical care in the community. Given the fiscal pressures facing BOP, as well as the rest of the government, it is critical that the agency focus its efforts on factors within its sphere of influence to ensure the prudent use of resources.

In many ways, BOP's efforts to understand and control its costs have been thwarted by limited data or limited applications of data already available. Although BOP recognizes the need for health care utilization data, and has identified a number of options for collecting these data, it has not yet assessed the most cost effective approach for obtaining such data. Conducting a cost-effectiveness analysis of the competing alternative solutions, and taking steps toward implementation of the most effective solution, would allow BOP to dedicate its resources judiciously.

Further, while BOP has engaged other federal agencies to leverage purchasing power, it has not consistently collected and analyzed health care spending data across its institutions. Conducting a comprehensive spend analysis could help BOP identify additional strategic sourcing opportunities to acquire medical goods and services more efficiently.

In addition, BOP has undertaken various initiatives to control health costs but does not have assurance that these initiatives are achieving their cost control aim because it has not evaluated its initiatives on a regular basis. BOP has also not incorporated certain elements of sound planning into its strategic health care plans, including identifying a means to measure progress toward goals and objectives and a means to measure effectiveness of activities. BOP also has not identified the resources and investments needed to implement its initiatives, an additional element of sound planning that can help ensure successful implementation. By incorporating these sound planning elements, BOP could enhance its planning and implementation efforts before expending resources, better positioning itself for success as it aims to control health care costs.

Finally, when BOP sets out to make decisions about how to shift or consolidate resources—as it does when conducting its mission analyses—it does not document its analyses and findings to support its recommendations for decisions about resources. Strengthening this process would enhance its internal control system and better support the decisions it makes.

Recommendations for Executive Action

We recommend that the Director of BOP take the following five actions:

1) To better understand the available opportunities for collecting inmate health care utilization data, BOP should conduct a cost-effectiveness analysis of potential solutions, and take steps toward implementation of the most effective solution.
2) To better understand the available opportunities for controlling health care costs, BOP should implement its guidance to conduct "spend analyses" of BOP's health care spending, using data sources already available.
3) To determine the actual or likely effectiveness of its ongoing or planned health care cost control initiatives, BOP should evaluate the extent to which its initiatives achieve their cost control aim.
4) To enhance its strategic planning for and implementation of health care cost control efforts, BOP should incorporate elements of a sound planning approach and
   - establish a means of measuring progress toward and effectiveness of its activities for its current strategic objectives and goals related to controlling health care costs; and
   - identify the resources and investments necessary for implementation of its planned health care cost control initiatives.
5) To improve the reliability and utility of its Federal Medical Center mission analyses, BOP should document the analyses and findings that underlie its recommendations.

Agency Comments and Our Evaluation

We provided a draft of this report to DOJ for review and comment. DOJ did not provide official written comments to include in this report.

However, in an e-mail received on June 20, 2017, a DOJ official stated that BOP concurred with all five recommendations.

BOP also provided technical comments, which we incorporated as appropriate.

We are sending copies of this report to the Attorney General, selected congressional committees, and other interested parties. In addition, this report is also available at no charge on the GAO website at http://www.gao.gov.

If you or your staff have any further questions about this report, please contact me at (202) 512-8777 or goodwing@gao.gov. Contact points for our Offices of Congressional Relations and Public Affairs may be found on the last page of this report. Key contributions to this reported are listed in appendix IV.

Gretta L. Goodwin
Director, Homeland Security and Justice Issues

Appendix I: Objectives, Scope, and Methodology

Our objectives for this report were to examine: (1) how much the Bureau of Prisons (BOP) has obligated for inmate health care from fiscal years 2009 through 2016 and the factors that affect BOP's costs, (2) the extent to which BOP has data available to understand and help control its costs, and (3) the initiatives BOP has identified and implemented to help control health care costs and the extent to which BOP has effectively planned its health care cost control efforts.

To examine how much BOP has obligated for inmate health services over the past 8 fiscal years and the factors that have affected BOP's costs, we interviewed officials from BOP's Administration Division, Health Services Division (HSD), Psychology Services Branch, and Field Acquisition Office, as well as officials within BOP's six regional offices and at the 10 individual BOP institutions we visited, to understand why obligations have changed over time and the factors that have impacted those changes.[72] We selected the 10 BOP institutions to visit based in part on factors that both BOP and existing research indicated could be affecting costs, as well as other factors that allowed for variation in our sample. These factors included the institutions' medical care levels; their total and per capita medical services costs; the characteristics of the institutions' population, including gender and percentage of inmates age 55 or older; and geography.[73] The 10 institutions we visited encompassed all four medical care levels, had a range of per capita medical services costs from low to high, included both male and female populations, housed lower and higher percentages of inmates age 55 or older, were located in remote and metropolitan areas, and covered all six of BOP's regions. Although not generalizable, the visits provided important insight into how different institution and inmate characteristics impact costs. In addition, we reviewed key documents, such as BOP's Congressional Budget Justifications for fiscal years 2009 through 2018, BOP's Annual Financial Statements, and the Department of Justice's Financial Management Information System Sub-Object Classification (SOC) Code Guide.[74]

We also analyzed BOP obligation data from fiscal year 2009 to 2016 on medical services, psychology services, drug and sex offender treatment

---

[72] The institutions we visited were United States Penitentiary Atwater, Federal Correctional Complex Beaumont, Federal Correctional Complex Butner, Federal Medical Center Carswell, Federal Correctional Complex Coleman, Federal Correctional Institution Fort Dix, Federal Correctional Institution Fort Worth, Federal Medical Center Lexington, Metropolitan Correctional Center New York, and Federal Medical Center Rochester. At the time of our visit, Fort Worth was a Federal Correctional Institution, but later became a Federal Medical Center.

[73] We computed the average age of inmates for each individual institution and calculated the percentage of inmates age 55 or older. We picked the age of 55 based on discussions with BOP officials, subject matter experts, and on academic and trade organization papers, who noted that 55 and older is generally the age at which inmates experience health problems related to aging. We then aggregated this information for BOP overall.

[74] Federal agencies use SOC Code Guides to standardize budgetary information. SOC codes define the nature of services or articles obligated.

programs, and medical staff training.[75] We included 8 years of obligations data in order to observe trends over time in health care costs. We decided to be inclusive of all categories of health care that are considered to be essential to treating health, which includes mental health and substance use disorder treatment. To determine the per capita obligations, we divided the total obligation by the inmate population at the end of each fiscal year. To adjust the per capita obligations for inflation, we used fiscal year 2016 as the baseline and adjusted each prior year to 2016 dollars by the Bureau of Economic Analysis and the IHS Global Insight Outlook inflation factor.[76] To better understand the composition of medical services obligations, we analyzed the breakout of these obligations by SOC code. Specifically, we used the SOC Code Guide to understand the various codes and how they could be grouped. We settled on five overarching categories: (1) salaries and benefits for medical staff, as well as related employee expenses, such as work travel; (2) outside medical care, which includes contractual medical services provided both inside and outside of BOP institutions by non-BOP medical staff; (3) supplies and materials, which includes pharmaceutical purchasing and other materials used in the provision of health services; (4) equipment of a durable nature, such as tools and implements, machinery, and information technology hardware; and (5) other, for all obligations that did not fit into the other categories, such as transportation of things, rent, communications, utilities, printing, and insurance claims.

To better understand the changes in pharmaceutical obligations over our time period, and what illnesses were impacting those obligations, we analyzed BOP's list of top 50 medications for fiscal years 2009 through 2016, and compared the medications to the U.S. National Library of Medicine's MedlinePlus list of drugs and supplements in order to determine the uses.[77] We compiled a list of medications used to treat

[75] BOP includes dental services as part of medical services.

[76] IHS Global Insight is a firm that provides comprehensive economic and financial information on countries, regions, and industries.

[77] MedlinePlus, produced by the National Library of Medicine, is the National Institutes of Health's web site that contains extensive information on prescription and nonprescription drugs, in addition to information on over 1,000 diseases and conditions.

hepatitis C, cancer, human immunodeficiency virus/acquired immune deficiency syndrome (HIV/AIDS), and psychotropic medications, which are generally used to treat mental illness. The remaining medications were used to treat a variety of illnesses, or were too few to create a category. We therefore created a category of other for the remaining medications. To assess the reliability of BOP's obligations and expenditures data, we (1) performed electronic data testing and looked for obvious errors in accuracy and completeness, and (2) interviewed agency officials knowledgeable about BOP's budget to determine the processes in place to ensure the integrity of the data. We determined that the data were sufficiently reliable for the purposes of this report. Finally, since geographic location may impact the provision or cost of inmate health care, we analyzed BOP institutions' proximity to hospitals.[78] To do this, we used geographic information services software to map the addresses of all BOP institutions, and verify how many hospitals were within a 20 mile radius of the institution.[79] We created four categories— institutions that had no hospitals within 20 miles, institutions that had 1 to 5 hospitals within 20 miles, institutions that had 6 to 10 hospitals with 20 miles, and institutions that had 11 or more hospitals within 20 miles.

To examine the extent to which BOP has data available to understand and help control its costs, the initiatives BOP has implemented and identified to help control health care costs, and how effectively BOP has planned and implemented these initiatives, we reviewed relevant BOP program statements. We conducted interviews with BOP officials from the Health Services, Reentry Services, and Information, Policy, and Public Affairs Divisions, as well as the Office of General Counsel in BOP's

---

78 For the purposes of our analysis, a hospital is defined as a building or building complex providing general medical or surgical inpatient care. It includes general hospitals, specialty hospitals (such as cancer, maternity, substance abuse, psychiatric, and rehabilitation hospitals). It does not include psychiatric or behavioral facilities that are not hospitals, long-term care medical centers or nursing homes, walk-in centers or outpatient clinics, imaging centers, medical doctors' offices, and rehabilitation centers.

79 BOP has 122 BOP-operated institutions, 39 of which are located in one of 15 Federal Correctional Complexes (FCC). FCCs are a cluster of institutions with different missions (for example, medical/mental health, pretrial, and holdover), which are located together. Because they are located together, for the purposes of this analysis we counted an FCC as one institution. When counting an FCC as one institution, there are 98 BOP institutions.

Central Office, given their responsibilities in this arena. We also interviewed officials from each of the six BOP regions and the Field Acquisition Office. Further, we reviewed current Office of Management and Budget (OMB) and BOP policies on cost-effectiveness analysis to analyze BOP's efforts to gather data. Additionally, for background on correctional health care costs and BOP health care, we reviewed articles and reports from various organizations, including the Congressional Budget Office, Congressional Research Service, and several academic and research institutes and interviewed researchers and economists from some of them to understand their methodologies and explore their findings. Further, we interviewed two correctional health clinicians from non-federal medical institutions due to their knowledge of the aging inmate population and telehealth. To determine the extent of available data on BOP health care costs, we searched the Federal Procurement Data System-Next Generation (FPDS-NG) for BOP contract actions by institution for fiscal years 2009 through 2015 and obtained pharmaceutical obligations data from BOP for that same period. Based on these steps, we determined the data were sufficiently reliable for the purposes of our reporting objective. In addition to interviews, to determine how well BOP's health care cost control planning mechanisms work, we obtained and reviewed selected portions of the annual BOP-wide strategic plans, the BOP's HSD Governing Board Meeting Minutes through 2015, and the HSD Strategic Plan for 2015 through 2019. To identify BOP's health care cost control efforts, their status of implementation, and the extent to which BOP had conducted cost estimates for each, we relied on the testimonial and documentary evidence the aforementioned BOP officials provided, reviewed previous GAO reports, Department of Justice (DOJ) Office of Inspector General (OIG) reports, and BOP Congressional Budget Justifications for fiscal years 2009 through 2018.[80] We summarized this information into a data collection instrument for verification by BOP

[80] See for example: GAO, *Bureau of Prisons: Information on Efforts and Potential Options to Save Costs*, GAO-14-821 (Washington, D.C.: Sept. 30, 2014). DOJ OIG, *The Federal Bureau of Prison's Efforts to Manage Inmate Health Care*, Audit Report 08-08 (Washington, D.C.: Feb. 2008); and *Follow-Up Audit of the Federal Bureau of Prisons' Efforts to Manage Inmate Health Care*, Audit Report 10-30 (Washington, D.C.: July 2010).

officials and requested additional data and supporting documentation for each. We reviewed the information BOP provided in the data collection instrument to identify missing or unclear information and resubmitted the data collection instrument for BOP's secondary verification. We also interviewed officials from DOJ OIG and DOJ's Justice Management Division[81] to discuss prior report recommendations on BOP health care costs. Further, at the 10 institutions we visited, we interviewed institution officials and observed health care programs and cost control efforts. We also requested and obtained several documents relating to the costs and cost savings of regional and institutional initiatives to control health care costs.

We conducted this performance audit from February 2016 to June 2017 in accordance with generally accepted government auditing standards. Those standards require that we plan and perform the audit to obtain sufficient, appropriate evidence to provide a reasonable basis for our findings and conclusions based on our audit objectives. We believe that the evidence obtained provides a reasonable basis for our findings and conclusions based on our audit objectives.

APPENDIX II: BUREAU OF PRISONS (BOP) INSTITUTIONS BY MEDICAL CARE LEVEL AS OF MARCH 2017

Medical care level[a]	Institution name[b]	Institution location
Care level 1		
	Atwater USP	Atwater, CA
	Bennettsville FCI	Bennettsville, SC
	Berlin FCI	Berlin, NH
	Big Sandy USP	Inez, KY
	Herlong FCI	Herlong, CA

[81] DOJ's Justice Management Division (JMD) provides DOJ with advice on policy for budget and financial management, program evaluation, auditing, personnel management and training, procurement, information processing and telecommunications, security and for all matters pertaining to organization, management, and administration. In 2012, JMD budget staff issued an assessment of BOP's method for procuring medical services and potential ways to reduce costs, including cost savings opportunities.

Appendix II. (Continued)

Medical care level[a]	Institution name[b]	Institution location
	Lee USP	Pennington Gap, VA
	Manchester FCI	Manchester, KY
	McDowell FCI	Welch, WV
	McKean FCI	Lewis Run, PA
	Mendota FCI	Mendota, CA
	Oxford FCI	Oxford, WI
	Pollock Medium FCI	Pollock, LA
	Pollock USP	Pollock, LA
	Ray Brook FCI	Ray Brook, NY
	Safford FCI	Safford, AZ
	Sandstone FCI	Sandstone, MN
	Three Rivers FCI	Three Rivers, TX
	Yankton FPC	Yankton, SD
	Yazoo City Low FCI	Yazoo City, MS
	Yazoo City Medium FCI	Yazoo City, MS
	Yazoo City USP	Yazoo City, MS
Total care level 1 institutions = 21		
Care level 2		
	Alderson FPC	Alderson, WV
	Aliceville FCI	Aliceville, AL
	Allenwood Low FCI	Allenwood, PA
	Allenwood Medium FCI	Allenwood, PA
	Allenwood USP	Allenwood, PA
	Ashland FCI	Ashland, KY
	Atlanta USP	Atlanta, GA
	Bastrop FCI	Bastrop, TX
	Beaumont Low FCI	Beaumont, TX
	Beaumont Med FCI	Beaumont, TX
	Beaumont USP	Beaumont, TX
	Beckley FCI	Beckley, WV
	Big Spring FCI	Big Spring, TX
	Brooklyn MDC	Brooklyn, NY
	Bryan FPC	Bryan, TX
	Butner Low FCI	Butner, NC
	Butner Medium I FCI	Butner, NC
	Butner Medium II FCI	Butner, NC
	Canaan USP	Waymart, PA
	Chicago MCC	Chicago, IL
	Coleman I USP	Sumterville, FL
	Coleman II USP	Sumterville, FL
	Coleman Low FCI	Sumterville, FL

Medical care level[a]	Institution name[b]	Institution location
	Coleman Medium FCI	Sumterville, FL
	Cumberland FCI	Cumberland, MD
	Danbury FCI	Danbury, CT
	Dublin FCI	Dublin, CA
	Duluth FPC	Duluth, MN
	Edgefield FCI	Edgefield, SC
	El Reno FCI	El Reno, OK
	Elkton FCI	Lisbon, OH
	Englewood FCI	Littleton, CO
	Estill FCI	Estill, SC
	Fairton FCI	Fairton, NJ
	Florence ADMAX USP	Florence, CO
	Florence FCI	Florence, CO
	Florence High USP	Florence, CO
	Forrest City Low FCI	Forrest City, AR
	Forrest City Medium FCI	Forrest City, AR
	Fort Dix FCI	Fort Dix, NJ
	Fort Worth FMC	Fort Worth, TX
	Gilmer FCI	Glenville, WV
	Greenville FCI	Greenville, IL
	Guaynabo MDC	Guaynabo, PR
	Hazelton FCI	Bruceton Mills, WV
	Hazelton USP	Bruceton Mills, WV
	Honolulu FDC	Honolulu, HI
	Houston FDC	Houston, TX
	Jesup FCI	Jesup, GA
	La Tuna FCI	Anthony, TX
	Leavenworth USP	Leavenworth, KS
	Lewisburg USP	Lewisburg, PA
	Lexington FMC	Lexington, KY
	Lompoc FCI	Lompoc, CA
	Lompoc USP	Lompoc, CA
	Loretto FCI	Loretto, PA
	Los Angeles MDC	Los Angeles, CA
	Marianna FCI	Marianna, FL
	Marion USP	Marion, IL
	McCreary USP	Pine Knot, KY
	Memphis FCI	Memphis, TN
	Miami FCI	Miami, FL
	Miami FDC	Miami, FL
	Milan FCI	Milan, MI
	Montgomery FPC	Montgomery, AL
	Morgantown FCI	Morgantown, WV
	New York MCC	New York, NY

Appendix II. (Continued)

Medical care level[a]	Institution name[b]	Institution location
	Oakdale I FCI	Oakdale, LA
	Oakdale II FCI	Oakdale, LA
	Oklahoma City FTC	Oklahoma City, OK
	Otisville FCI	Otisville, NY
	Pekin FCI	Pekin, IL
	Pensacola FPC	Pensacola, FL
	Petersburg Low FCI	Hopewell, VA
	Petersburg Medium FCI	Hopewell, VA
	Philadelphia FDC	Philadelphia, PA
	Phoenix FCI	Phoenix, AZ
	San Diego MCC	San Diego, CA
	Schuylkill FCI	Minersville, PA
	Seagoville FCI	Seagoville, TX
	Seatac FDC	Seattle, WA
	Sheridan FCI	Sheridan, OR
	Talladega FCI	Talladega, AL
	Tallahassee FCI	Tallahassee, FL
	Terminal Island FCI	San Pedro, CA
	Terre Haute FCI	Terre Haute, IN
	Terre Haute USP	Terre Haute, IN
	Texarkana FCI	Texarkana, TX
	Thomson Administrative USP	Thomson, IL
	Tucson FCI	Tucson, AZ
	Tucson USP	Tucson, AZ
	Victorville Medium I FCI	Victorville, CA
	Victorville Medium II FCI	Victorville, CA
	Victorville USP	Victorville, CA
	Waseca FCI	Waseca, MN
	Williamsburg FCI	Salters, SC
Total care level 2 institutions = 96		
Care level 3		
	Allenwood Medium FCI	Allenwood, PA
	Allenwood USP	Allenwood, PA
	Butner FMC	Butner, NC
	Butner Low FCI	Butner, NC
	Butner Medium I FCI	Butner, NC
	Butner Medium II FCI	Butner, NC
	Carswell FMC	Fort Worth, TX
	Coleman I USP	Sumterville, FL
	Coleman II USP	Sumterville, FL
	Coleman Medium FCI	Sumterville, FL

Medical care level[a]	Institution name[b]	Institution location
	Devens FMC	Ayer, MA
	Fort Worth FMC	Fort Worth, TX
	Lexington FMC	Lexington, KY
	Rochester FMC	Rochester, MN
	Springfield MCFP	Springfield, MO
	Terminal Island FCI	San Pedro, CA
	Terre Haute FCI	Terre Haute, IN
	Terre Haute USP	Terre Haute, IN
	Tucson USP	Tucson, AZ
	Victorville USP	Victorville, CA
Total care level 3 institutions = 20		
Care level 4		
	Butner FMC	Butner, NC
	Carswell FMC	Fort Worth, TX
	Devens FMC	Ayer, MA
	Fort Worth FMC	Fort Worth, TX
	Lexington FMC	Lexington, KY
	Rochester FMC	Rochester, MN
	Springfield MCFP	Springfield, MO
Total care level 4 institutions = 7		

Legend:

FCC refers to Federal Correctional Complex

FCI refers to Federal Correctional Institution

FDC refers to Federal Detention Center

FMC refers to Federal Medical Center.

FPC refers to Federal Prison Camp

FTC refers to Federal Transfer Center.

MCC refers to Metropolitan Correctional Center

MCFP refers to Medical Center for Federal Prisoners

MDC refers to Metropolitan Detention Center.

USP refers to U.S. Penitentiary

Source: BOP. | GAO-17-379.

[a]BOP classifies both institutions and inmates by care level. BOP does not define the criterion for the institution care level but rather bases it on the medical resources available to meet the needs of inmates of a particular care level. Generally, institutions at each care level are designed to house mostly inmates at that designated medical and mental care level; however, inmates housed at every institution will be comprised of a mixture of care levels. According to BOP, factors that affect inmate care level variation includes changes in health status, proximity to family, separation from threat groups, security level, ongoing legal cases, or participation in residential treatment programs. No institution will have an inmate population composed of a given care level.

[b]Some institutions are categorized as two different care levels (i.e., care level 1 and 2, or 2 and 3, or 3 and 4) and therefore are double counted in this table. Additionally, some institutions are complexes made up of two or more institutions. The institutions within the complexes are counted separately.

APPENDIX III: BUREAU OF PRISONS (BOP) FEDERAL MEDICAL CENTERS

BOP has seven care level 4 institutions, also referred to as Federal Medical Centers (FMC), spread out throughout the United States.[82] The FMCs provide care to inmates in need of more advanced medical or mental health care. Following are descriptions for each FMC.

- FMC Butner (Butner, North Carolina) is part of an FCC and serves as a major medical and psychiatric referral center for male inmates. FMC Butner has all specialty areas of medicine and is the primary referral center for oncology, providing chemotherapy and radiation therapy. FMC Butner also manages a broad range of subacute and chronically ill inmates and has an orthopedic surgery program available. Dialysis services are provided on-site. Butner also has an extensive inpatient forensics program. As of May 2017, there were 927 inmates at FMC Butner.
- FMC Carswell (Fort Worth, Texas) serves as the major medical and psychiatric referral center for female inmates. All specialty areas of medicine are available through in-house staff and community-based consultant specialists. As of May 2017, there were 1,171 inmates at FMC Carswell.
- FMC Devens (Devens, Massachusetts) serves both medical and mental health care needs for male inmates. All specialty areas of medicine are available through in-house staff and community-based consultant specialists. Additional services provided include dialysis treatment for inmates with end-stage renal failure. As of May 2017, there were 956 inmates at FMC Devens.
- FMC Fort Worth (Fort Worth, Texas) officially began its medical center mission on December 7, 2016. When fully operational,

[82] Six of the medical referral centers are named Federal Medical Center (FMC) and one is named United States Medical Center for Federal Prisoners. According to BOP, there is no salient difference in the medical mission for the seven institutions and therefore all can be referred to as FMCs.

FMC Fort Worth will serve both medical and mental health needs of male inmates. The institution will expand from 36 to 72 medical beds having 24-hour nursing care, and will include a 21-bed inpatient forensics unit and a care level 3 Mental Health Step Down Unit Program.[83] BOP anticipates that all necessary building renovations and hiring of medical center staff will be completed within 24 months of its formal conversion to a medical center mission. As of May 2017, there were 1,492 inmates at FMC Fort Worth.

- FMC Lexington (Lexington, Kentucky) serves male inmates. All specialty areas of medicine are available by in-house staff and community-based consultant specialists. FMC Lexington serves as the primary referral center for inmates with most types of leukemia and lymphoma, and performs outpatient forensic studies. As of May 2017, there were 1,356 inmates at FMC Lexington.
- FMC Rochester (Rochester, Minnesota) serves as a major medical and mental health referral center for male inmates. FMC Rochester is the primary referral center for inmates with end-stage liver disease and advanced HIV infection, as well as other infectious diseases requiring long-term management. FMC Rochester provides extensive psychiatric and psychology services, including inpatient psychiatry services and forensic studies. As of May 2017, there were 665 inmates at FMC Rochester.
- U.S. Medical Center for Federal Prisoners (MCFP) Springfield (Springfield, Missouri) serves as a major medical and psychiatric referral center for male inmates. MCFP Springfield provides all specialty areas of medicine through in-house staff and community-based consultant specialists, and is the primary referral center for high security inmates. The institution maintains extensive psychiatric and psychological services, to include inpatient

[83] The Mental Health Step Down Unit Program is a residential treatment program offering an intermediate level of care for inmates with serious mental illnesses. The program is specifically designed to serve inmates who do not require inpatient treatment, but lack the skills to function in a general population setting.

forensic studies. It is the major kidney dialysis center for the BOP. As of May 2017, there were 1,031 inmates at MCFP Springfield.

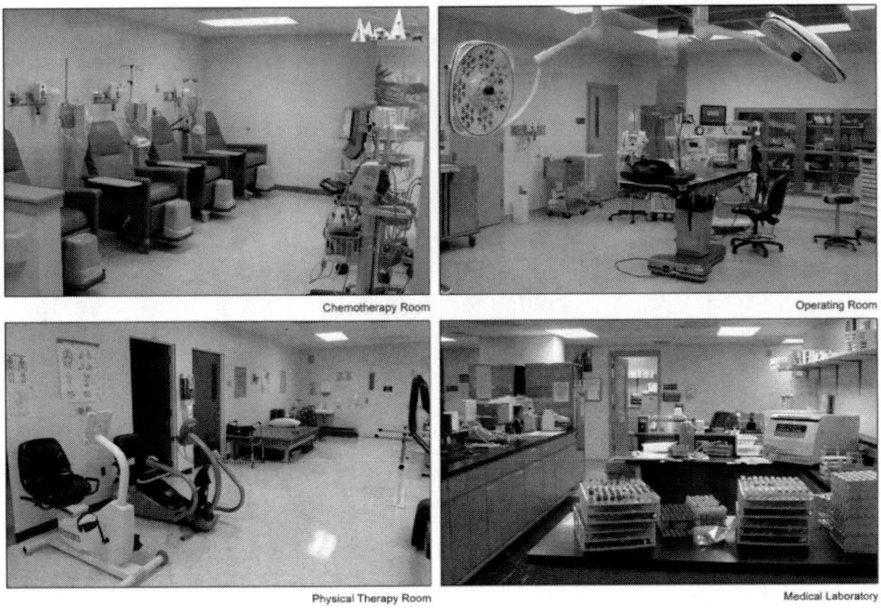

Source: BOP. | GAO-17-379.

Note: These images represent various health care facilities at BOP institutions. They are not necessarily reflective of the facilities at all BOP institutions, which may differ based on medical care level and available resources.

Figure 8. Selected Images of Health Services Facilities and Equipment at Bureau of Prisons' (BOP) Federal Medical Centers.

INDEX

C

D

E

F

G

H

I

N

O

P